Inferences of Patients' Pain
and
Psychological Distress

Studies of Nursing Behaviors

Joel R. Davitz, Ph.D., received his bachelor's degree from the University of Illinois and his doctoral degree from Columbia University. Since 1955 he has been on the faculty of Teachers College, Columbia University, and is currently Professor of Psychology and Education. Author of *Language of Emotion, The Communication of Emotional Meaning*, and co-author of several other books, Dr. Davitz has published extensively in professional journals. He served as co-principal investigator of the research project, Nurses' Inferences of Physical Pain and Psychological Distress. In addition, Dr. Davitz has served as consultant on a wide variety of nursing projects and as participant in nursing education workshops and conferences.

Lois Leiderman Davitz, Ph.D., received her bachelor's degree from the University of Michigan and master's and doctoral degrees from Columbia University. She has been associated with the department of nursing education at Teachers College, Columbia University, since 1964. She was co-principal investigator of the research project, Nurses' Inferences of Physical Pain and Psychological Distress. Author of *Interpersonal Processes in Nursing: Case Histories, The Psychiatric Patient: Case Histories,* and co-author of several other books, Dr. Davitz has written many articles on research and nursing in professional journals. In addition to her work in the United States, she has been lecturer and coordinator of nursing conferences and workshops in various parts of Africa.

Inferences of Patients' Pain
and
Psychological Distress

Studies of Nursing Behaviors

Joel R. Davitz, Ph.D.
Lois Leiderman Davitz, Ph.D.

Springer Publishing Company
New York

Springer Publishing Company, Inc.
200 Park Avenue South
New York, New York 10003

   82 83 84 / 10 9 8 7 6 5 4 3 2

Library of Congress Cataloging in Publication Data

Davitz, Joel Robert.
   Inferences of patients' pain and psychological
distress.

   Bibliography: p.
   Includes index.
   1. Nursing—Psychological aspects. 2. Pain—
Psychological aspects. 3. Pain—Nursing. 4. Nurse
and patient. 5. Suffering. 6. Inference (Logic).
I. Davitz, Lois Jean, joint author. II. Title. [DNLM: 1. Attitude
of health personnel. 2. Nurse-patient relations.
3. Nursing care—Psychology. WY87 D263i]
RT86.D37   610.73'01'9   80-23830
ISBN 0-8261-3360-6
ISBN 0-8261-3361-4 (pbk.)

Printed in the United States of America

Contents

Part Four
Changes in Nurses' Beliefs

Part Five
Beliefs and Behaviors

Part Six
Summary and Discussion

Foreword

When the Doctors Davitz asked if I would be willing to write a foreword for this book, I responded that I would be delighted to do so—for several reasons. First, this book, unlike so many others marketed for nurses, addresses a subject matter that has *real* significance for nurses and is central to nursing practice. Suffering and the remedy thereof is central to any concept of nursing which perceives the nurse as caregiver, sustainer, and one who supports the patient through an illness experience. Clearly, research which reflects upon suffering, its interpretation, or its management is crucial for the nursing discipline. The impressive collection of research projects in this book concerning suffering clearly contributes information to this critical subject.

Second, I am pleased to participate in this book—if only in a small way—because it illustrates the possibility of doing creative and sound research concerning the nursing domain. Too much so-called nursing research is abstracted from the clinical domain and carried out under circumstances so far removed that application of findings to the clinical area is questionable. Results of the research projects in this book, however, are directly relevant to clinical nursing and medical practice and education.

Finally, this book, unlike much nursing research, does not merely confirm the obvious. As a mystery fan, I found myself caught up in many of the studies—anxiously awaiting the outcomes. And many of those outcomes had the surprise of a good mystery.

As to the substance of the research, the studies move from one perspective to another, continually increasing the reader's knowledge of the total subject matter of suffering. The study, therefore, is a remarkable effort at the single concept (in this case, suffering) approach to theory-building.

The first set of studies explores nurses themselves and their own beliefs about suffering as it relates to certain characteristics of the patient. In this set of studies, the researchers devise a basic tool which attempts to differentiate perspectives on suffering according to severity and type of illness, including both psychological and physical illnesses. The tool attempts to differentiate (1) classes of illness: cardiovascular, traumatic, psychiatric, cancerous, and infectious; and (2) degree of severity: mild, moderate, or severe. One illness/state is selected to exemplify each cell in this 3 × 5 table. One may argue that these cells say more about the individually selected illness/state in the cell than they say about the particular class or severity of illness. For example, the identity of "possible leukemia" for the moderate-cancer cell causes some irregularities in response. (Nurses clearly recognized the suffering related to an unknown diagnosis as being virtually equal to that associated with a known and undesired diagnosis.) Nevertheless, whether the tool reflects judgments about classes, severity, or specific illness/states, it still serves as a useful mechanism by which to make comparisons among perceptions of nurses. Responses to the tool are clearly differentiated according to characteristics of the nurses themselves.

While I would like to relay immediately all the fascinating results of this section of the research, that would be like giving away the ending of a good mystery. Let me, therefore, only present the least surprising finding: that a nurse's perception of suffering relates to his or her own personal past experience of (or lack of experience of) pain and suffering.

The next section of the book takes the reader a step further by differentiating nursing groups according to cross-cultural factors. Not only are different ethnic groups of nurses found to perceive suffering differently, but they are found to perceive suffering differently for different ethnic groups of patients. The interplay of these two ethnicity factors—patients and nurses—is intriguing. Ironically, many nurses are found to infer that the least suffering takes place among certain cultures whose own nurse members classify themselves as suffering more intensely than other groups. These studies present evidence of ironic misconceptions of suffering.

Further, evidence is presented that many nurses view stoics not as better maskers of suffering, but as suffering less than others. Some evidence in these studies would indicate, conversely, that stoicism may mask greater, not lesser, degrees of suffering. Hence, in some cases, nurses are found to have the least empathy for the patients who most need it. Again, I will preserve the mystery, and let the readers discover these cross-cultural factors for themselves.

After having collected and presented much quantitative data, the Doctors Davitz now illustrate their ability to handle qualitative data also. They sensitively describe the empathic nurse, tracing those elements of character, experience, and education which impact upon empathic development. Insights abound here for student selection and education.

The researchers did not stop here but went on to relate empathy—or the lack of it—to nursing behaviors. As a former nursing service administrator, I was excited to see these nursing behaviors further related to the situational context in which the nurse was practicing. Hence the authors take the final step of relating the theoretical concept (suffering) to extant nurse behavior.

Here we have a research work which leaves the reader with the same sense of completion as a good novel, having moved from a concept, to the explication of implicit belief systems, and on to the impaction upon extant nursing practices.

Not the least of this study is the sensitive and insightful interpretation of data by the researchers. This interpretation escapes the usual short-sighted valuation which often cuts off further thought and inquiry. For example, the authors suspend judgment and explore the mechanism by which nurses distance themselves from the patient's suffering. Rather than offering unthinking censure, they explore the nurse's need for distancing, and find that this need may be greatest in the most sensitive nurse. The authors present an insightful analysis of the dilemma created for the nurse by mutual needs for sensitivity and for distance.

Most important, the Doctors Davitz raise some real nursing problems—such as the misfit between the psychological mechanisms taught to students as means of relief and the realities of their contacts with patients. Simply put, many of our "remedies" are just not applicable in the given contextual setting of the acute care hospital.

The Davitz team also discovers some major deficits that occur in nursing's educational system, such as the fact that nurse students are being sensitized to psychological suffering but desensitized to physical pain. Insightful discussions of problems such as this are included in the final sections of this book.

In summary, it is seldom that the nurse reader finds careful, valid research on a significant topic, with practical applications, presented in a clear and interesting manner. This book succeeds on all counts.

Barbara J. Stevens, R.N., Ph.D.

Acknowledgments

We would like to express our profound appreciation to the many individuals who contributed so much to the successful completion of the various studies concerned with *Inferences of Patients' Pain and Psychological Distress: Studies of Nursing Behaviors.* We wish to thank the directors of nursing of the forty-five cooperating hospitals. Their outstanding cooperation, invaluable suggestions, and continual support were extremely important to all phases of the investigation. We are deeply indebted to the eight thousand professional nurses in the United States who were actively involved in one or several of the studies. We also want to thank the fourteen hundred nurses from Japan, Korea, Thailand, Israel, Uganda, Belgium, Nigeria, England, Nepal, India, Puerto Rico, and Taiwan for their participation in the cross-cultural phases of the research. To these individuals and to countless others who were involved at various stages of this research, we extend our respect and deep sense of gratitude.

This research was supported by Grant No. NU 00496 from the Nursing Research Branch, Division of Nursing, Department of Health, Education and Welfare.

Joel R. Davitz, Ph.D.
Lois Leiderman Davitz, Ph.D.

Research Assistants:
Yasuko Higuchi, B.S.N., R.N., Ed.D.
Elizabeth Vecchione, B.S.N., R.N., M.A.
Geraldine Verrassi, B.S.N., R.N., M.Ed.

Part One

The Research Problem

1
A Theoretical Framework

In recent years, nurses have assumed an increasingly wide range of administrative, educational, and therapeutic responsibilities. Nevertheless, caring for patients who experience suffering represents a central aspect of nursing practice. Although nursing educators and theorists have recognized the significance of understanding patients' suffering, there have been relatively few systematic investigations focused on nurses' perceptions and reactions to patients' suffering. A number of previous studies have considered various methods of reducing pain and psychological distress, but few investigations have been directly concerned with nurses' reactions to patients that are suffering and need some form of comforting care. For one reason or another, nursing research has practically bypassed an essential part of the nursing process. Indeed, a few studies have investigated cues of patient distress, but these investigations represent only a bare beginning of a line of research concerned with a central aspect of nursing.

The present research, therefore, was designed to increase our understanding of nurses' reactions to the suffering of others. The initial phase of this research focused on individual and group differences among nurses in their beliefs about suffering. Based on these investigations, the research considered the central variable, reactions to suffering, in relation to effectiveness of nursing behaviors, providing a direct empirical linkage to nursing practice. Finally, shifting from the hospital setting to schools of nursing, changes in students' beliefs about patients' suffering were investigated over the course of nursing education. The results of this research add to our knowledge of nurses and the nursing process, and contribute to the development of nursing theory as well as to the improvement of nursing practice and education.

Previous Research

There are countless essays and books in the nursing literature that emphasize the nurse's role in the relief of patient suffering (see, Berblinger, 1959; Duff & Hollingshead, 1968; Johnson & Martin, 1958; Jourard, 1960; McCaffery &

Moss, 1967; Orlando, 1961). Indeed, this function is generally recognized as central to the professional role of the nurse. Congruent with this point of view are the results reported by Hammond (1966a, 1966b, 1967), who studied the kinds of tasks confronting nurses. Among other findings, Hammond reported that the most frequent cause for patients' summoning nurses is complaint of pain. In another survey of hospital patients, Dichter (1954) found that various aspects of psychological distress motivate most patients' complaints, and Skipper (1965) reported that patients most frequently wanted nurses to provide information or relief from pain and psychological distress. Thus, the theoretical, professional, and research literature is consistent in underscoring the response to patient suffering as a primary dimension of nursing.

Perceiving the Suffering of Others

There has been relatively little research focused specifically on nurses' assessments of patients' pain. However, Sullivan (1974) studies the cues nurses report they use in evaluating patients' pain. These cues include patients' verbalizations describing their pain and requesting relief, the nurses' interpretations of the patients' context, and objective nursing observations. Although a substantial minority of nurses (approximately 40 percent) emphasized the importance of verbal cues, an equal percentage of nurses ranked verbal cues as least important. Thus, there appears to be no generally shared consensus among nurses about which cues are most important in assessing patients' pain.

McCaffery (1972), who was concerned with the cues used to assess another person's pain, suggested that behaviors in response to pain might be classified into eight categories: (1) physiological manifestations, (2) verbal statements, (3) vocal behaviors, (4) facial expressions, (5) body movements, (6) physical contact, (7) general response to the environment, and (8) patterns of handling pain. While McCaffery emphasized a multidimensional approach to assessing pain, other writers such as Keele (1975), Loan and Dundie (1967), and Lasagna (1960) focus primarily on verbal methods of assessment.

Cues of distress were investigated by Johnson, Johnson, and Dumas (1970) who focused on variables such as pulse rate, blood pressure, and judgments of restlessness. In contrast, Graham and Conley (1971) concluded that, among preoperative patients, verbal statements were the most useful indicators of anxiety. In any event, Newton, Hunt, McDowell, and Hanken (1966) found that nurses were far more likely to react to patients' verbal reports of pain than to nonverbal signals indicative of distress. In another study of pain signals manifested by patients, Bochnak (1961) found that patients' complaints reflect a variety of underlying psychological problems, and Elder (1963) reported that patients frequently had great difficulty in expressing their emotional needs verbally. Recognizing the verbal limitations of many patients, Parisen, Rich, and Jackson (1969) developed a scale designed for the report of subjective stress, suggesting that this procedure might be useful, especially with patients who are unable to verbalize their discomfort.

Individual Differences in Pain Perception

Considerable research has been focused on the perception and measurement of pain (see Beecher, 1959; Melzack, 1961). Of particular importance to the proposed project is a line of investigation by Jacox, though at the present time only a preliminary report of this investigation is available. Specifically, Jacox and Stewart (1973) report a study of psychosocial factors related to type of pain, defined as short-term (for example, patients who had undergone appendectomies), long-term (patients with rheumatoid arthritis), and progressive (patients with metastatic cancer involving the abdominal region). Using the Eysenck *Personality Inventory,* the *Problems Inventory,* and a modification of Melzack's pain description questionnaire, Jacox and Stewart found that type of pain was related to extraversion and neuroticism as well as to the amount and kinds of problems associated with patients' illnesses. Obviously, this research has important implications for nurses' reactions to patients' suffering, for it suggests that patients' recognition and expression of feelings of pain are a function of psychological factors such as extraversion-introversion, neuroticism, and anxiety. Jacox's investigation and the present research thus represent complementary approaches to essentially the same general problem area, with Jacox focusing on the important issue of psychosocial factors related to the *patients'* experiences and reports of pain, and the present research focusing on nurses' reactions to patients' pain and psychological distress. Both lines of research, of course, converge in terms of implications for the development of nursing theory and the improvement of nursing practice based on the complementary knowledge gained from these related lines of investigation.

Psychosocial Factors in Pain Perception

The importance of psychosocial variables such as fear, experimental instructions, previous experience, and group membership has been investigated by researchers such as Gelfand (1964), Lambert, Libman, and Poser (1960), Hall and Stride (1954), Clark (1974), and Blitz and Dinnerstein (1968). Beecher (1957, 1959) suggests that the experience of suffering in relation to pain does not only depend on the noxious stimulus eliciting the physical sensation, but also is influenced by psychosocial factors such as the individual's cultural background and the immediate situation in which the noxious stimulus is encountered.

Meehan, Stoll, and Hardy (1954) did not find consistent differences in pain threshold among groups of Alaskan Indians, Eskimos, and Caucasians. However, Chapman (1944) and Chapman and Jones (1944) found that Southern Negro, Russian, Jewish, and Italian subjects have lower pain tolerance than Caucasian Americans with Northern European backgrounds. In a related study, Zborowski (1969) compared reactions to pain among Italian, Jewish, and "Old American" patients and found quite distinctive and different patterns of response characterizing these three groups. Similarly, Sternbach and Tursky (1965) found differences in attitudes toward pain reported by American "Yankee," Irish, Jewish, and Italian subjects.

Sex Differences in Pain Perception

Although investigators such as Critchley (1934), Hall and Stride (1954), and Kennard (1952) reported that women are more sensitive than men to pain, other investigators such as Clausen and King (1950), Hardy, Wolff, and Goodell (1952), and Swartz (1951) report no consistent differences between men and women in pain sensitivity. However, as suggested by Notermans and Tophoff (1975), studies of sex differences in pain sensitivity are complicated by cultural expectations that men in comparison to women should be "more tolerant of pain."

Reducing Patient Suffering

By far the most frequently reported topic in this general area concerns various methods of reducing patient suffering, considered either in terms of pain or psychological distress. Although this line of investigation is somewhat tangential to the immediate aims of the research, it may be useful to consider some illustrative studies in this area in terms of a general background for the research reported here. An eventual aim, of course, for both nursing theory and practice is the integration of research concerned with reactions to pain and psychological distress and studies of the reduction of patient suffering.

A substantial number of studies have focused on various kinds of communication variables. By and large, these studies report positive results. For example, Dumas and Leonard (1963) found that, if a nurse spent time talking with and listening to a patient prior to surgery, the patient tended to show less distress after surgery. Putt (1970) found that this kind of verbal interaction also reduced pain and stress among peptic ulcer patients; and McBride (1967), Bochnak (1961), Moss and Meyer (1966), Jarasuh, Rhymes, and Leonard (1965), and Kyle (1964) found similar results with a wide variety of patients under different hospital conditions. Although a few studies in this area have reported inconclusive or null results, (Barron, 1964; Chambers and

Price, 1967; Cohen, 1970; Diers, Schmidt, McBride, and Kette, 1972), the bulk of research supports the general hypothesis that communication between nurse and patient can serve to reduce both pain and psychological distress, though the nature of effective communication has not been empirically described in much detail.

Several studies have considered the effects of giving information to the patient. Healy (1968), for example, reported that preoperative information about what to expect, and so on, resulted in reduced postoperative stress; in contrast, Keller (1965) reported that patients who were given information by nurses manifested greater anxiety than patients who did not receive information. Focusing on somewhat more general variables, Hays and Larson (1963) and Hays (1966) found that both group and individual instruction relevant to their illnesses does indeed reduce the problems encountered by many patients.

Very little systematic work has been done on nonverbal means of reducing stress. Hallstrom (1968) found that babies held during injections cried less than babies who were not held, but DeAugustinis, Isani, and Kumler (1963), examining various nonverbal approaches to reducing anxiety, suggest that touch may increase patient anxiety, and the use of touch must be based on an assessment of the individual patient's needs.

The Interpretation of Pain

Copp (1973, 1974) investigated the ways in which patients interpreted suffering. Some viewed the experience as a challenge, others as an enemy, a weakness, punishment, loss, or damage. Copp interpreted her findings in terms of patients' philosophical orientations and beliefs and considered the congruency of patients' and nurses' beliefs in relation to the accuracy of nurses' assessments of patients' pain.

Merskey (1968) has emphasized the communication process in viewing pain. He suggests that patients' expressions of pain may be interpreted as messages referring to bodily symptoms, as requests for help, or as symbolic forms of aggression which may serve to expiate guilt.

Changes during Nursing Education

One aspect of the present research concerns changes in students' beliefs about suffering over the course of nursing education. Relatively few studies have systematically investigated changes in attitudes, values, and beliefs among nursing students. Perhaps the most attention has been paid to changes in attitudes toward death. Golub and Reznikaff (1971), for example, compared the attitudes of 82 practicing nurses and 70 first-year students. Using a multiple choice questionnaire dealing with concepts, fears, and attitudes about death, these researchers report differences between graduate and student nurses primarily in terms of the graduates' recognition of psychological factors associated with death, autopsy, and treatment of the seriously ill. On the basis of their results Golub and Reznikaff suggest that nurses acquire common attitudes early in their professional careers, and these attitudes will tend to remain stable over fairly long periods of time.

In a related study of changes in nursing students' attitudes toward the dying patient, Yeaworth, Kapp and Winget (1974) found that seniors, in comparison to freshmen, showed a greater acceptance of feelings, more open communication, and broader flexibility in relation to dying patients and their families. Similarly, Lester, Getty, and Kneisl (1974), comparing the views of undergraduate nursing students, graduates, and nursing faculty found that fears of death decreased with increased education.

Tapping somewhat more general attitudes, Moody (1973) studied attitudes of cynicism and humanitarianism among first-year nursing students, senior students, and staff nurses. No significant differences were found for cynicism. However, the author reports some decrease in humanitarianism between freshman and senior years, and a slight increase between the senior year and later practice.

Schmid and Schmid (1973) investigated nursing students' attitudes toward the alcoholic, comparing the attitudes of freshman nursing students with the attitudes of the same students measured over two years later. These investigators found that the students' attitudes toward the alcoholic remained essentially the same throughout the two-year period.

In a study of value changes among nursing students, May and Ilardi (1973) administered the Allport-Vernon-Lindzey *Study of Values* several times during a three-year nursing program. They report an increase in aesthetic values over the course of the program, a decrease in religious values, and no change in other values.

Nikkari (1969) studied freshman-to-senior personality changes among nursing students and female liberal arts students. In general, both nursing and liberal arts students moved toward more liberal attitudes as seniors; the nursing students, in comparison to the liberal arts students, were more conservative, more restrictive, more interested in practical affairs, and less tolerant of ambiguity. Stein (1969), using the *Edwards Personal Preference Schedule,* compared the needs of nursing students as sophomores and seniors. These students over the course of their education showed an increased need for social activities, change, and autonomy, with some decrease in need for nurturance and deference.

Nurses' Reactions to Suffering

Previous studies reported by Davitz and Pendleton (1969a, b, c, & d), Baer, Davitz, and Lieb (1970), Lenburg, Glass, and Davitz (1970), and Lenburg, Burnside, and Davitz (1970) investigated the relation between reactions to suffering and variables such as national and cultural background of the nurse, clinical specialties, diagnosis of the patient, selected patient characteristics, mode of communication, level of nursing education, and professional identity. None of these studies can be considered conclusive; they are intended as pilot work for more comprehensive and systematic investigation represented by the present research. However, these earlier studies achieved three major results relevant to the present research: (1) they clearly indicated the potential value of this line of investigation for nursing theory and practice, (2) they provided a basis for identifying significant variables for further investigation, and (3) they established the usefulness of a format and procedure for the measurement of reactions to suffering. Thus, in a very meaningful way, these previous pilot studies prepared the groundwork for the present research.

A Conceptual Framework

Every patient experiences his or her own unique distress, and no one, of course, can directly perceive the suffering of another person. Suffering refers to subjective experience. Thus, any evaluation of the nature or degree of another person's suffering necessarily depends upon inference. Presumably, the inference is based on observed cues, but it is also influenced by one's characteristic inferential response to such cues. Thus, for example, given the same cues relevant to another person's distress, it would not be unreasonable to expect two observers to differ somewhat in the degree of suffering inferred.

Each of us has what might be viewed as an "implicit theory of suffering." This consists of a set of beliefs relevant to our judgments about the suffering of others. For example, one might believe that certain cues are associated with specific kinds of suffering: crying implies physical pain, while a trembling voice "means" psychological distress. At a more complex level, one might have certain beliefs related to characteristics of the person observed. For example, one might implicitly believe that when men cry, they are suffering more than when women cry. Or one might believe that, given the same observed conditions of illness, children suffer relatively more psychological distress than physical pain. These beliefs are usually not verbalized in any systematic way, and for the most part, they probably operate without the individual's explicit awareness. That is, one does not observe another person's behavior, refer explicitly to one's "belief system," and then make an inference about that person's suffering. Nevertheless, these implicit beliefs undoubtedly influence the inferences we make about another person's experiences.

A dimension of this belief system particularly important in the present research concerns the degree to which one tends to maximize or minimize reactions to the suffering of others. This is especially significant for nursing, since nursing care involves, to a large extent, responding to the suffering of patients. If two nurses respond to the same patient cues with inferences of different degrees of suffering, it is reasonable to expect that their nursing behaviors will also differ. And if nurses differ in their general tendencies to make such inferences about patients—some of them consistently maximizing the suffering of patients, some minimizing, and some who are consistently moderate in their inferences—it is reasonable to expect more or less generalized differences in their nursing behaviors.

Previous research reported by Davitz and Pendleton (1969a, b, c, & d), Baer, et al. (1970), Lenburg, Glass, and Davitz (1970), and Lenburg, Burnside, and Davitz (1970) does indeed support the assumption of individual differences among nurses concerning the degree of patient suffering they tend to infer. An important question, therefore, concerns the characteristics of nurses associated with these individual differences. In general, it seems reasonable to assume that one's own experiences of suffering are directly related to the inferences one makes about the suffering of others. If a person, for example, has experienced a great deal of pain in a given situation, it seems likely that that person will tend to infer a relatively high degree of pain in others observed in similar situations. Thus, variables concerned with the nurse's own experience of suffering are expected to be related to his or her reactions to patients' suffering. Several specific variables are suggested by this general hypothesis. Petrie (1967) found that individuals consistently differ from one another in their tendency to augment or reduce reactions to painful stimuli. In the psychological domain, Byrne (1961) has established a parallel finding with regards to psychological distress. Both Petrie and Byrne deal with more or less general personality characteristics or traits, but one would also expect a nurse's reactions to others to be related to his or her own experiences of suffering associated with personal illness. Directly related to these general considerations are Zborowski's findings regarding differences in reactions to pain among people in various subcultural groups (1969). If cultural variables make a difference in the nurse's own reactions to pain, one would expect these variables also to be related to inferences about the suffering of others.

Nursing offers opportunities to satisfy different kinds of interests, and nurses differ in the degree to which they value professional activities involving primarily technical skills and other professional skills involving relatively more humanistic concerns. A clearcut typology of nurses obviously is not implied by this distinction; most, if not all, nurses share both kinds of interests and values. Nevertheless, there are likely to be differences in the degree to which one interest is stronger than the other, and it seems reasonable to expect that technically oriented versus humanistically oriented nurses differ in their reactions to patients.

This difference in orientation is also reflected in the kinds of cues to which a nurse might attend in his or her interactions with patients. One nurse might pay particular attention to cues indicative of the patient's physiological functioning, while another nurse might be especially sensitive to cues relevant to the patient's emotional state. Assuming that suffering refers to the patient's affective experience (including pain as well as psychological distress in the psychological domain), one might expect that the degree to which one pays attention to, and presumably is concerned with, cues relevant to affect is related to reactions to the suffering of others.

In addition to the variables noted above, degree of inferred suffering may also be a function of the relationship between nurse and patient characteristics. For example, considering the subcultural backgrounds of nurse and patient, do white nurses tend to infer a different degree of suffering between white and black patients? Similarly, do black nurses tend to infer a different degree of suffering between white and black patients? Do relatively younger and older nurses differ in the degree of suffering they infer between younger and older patients?

Inferred suffering must also be considered in relation to nursing behaviors and effectiveness. It seems reasonable to expect that nurses who tend to infer a high degree of suffering among their patients differ both in the amount and nature of their interactions with patients, as well as in the effectiveness of their nursing care. However, previous theory, research, and clinical observations do not provide a basis for predicting the nature of these relationships. For example, at the outset of this research, there was no basis for identifying the "optimum" degree of sensitivity to patient suffering associated with effective care. Recent efforts in nursing education have been directed at the goal of sensitizing nurses to patients' feelings. Obviously, a nurse who is totally insensitive to his or her patients' feelings is not likely to provide very effective care, but there is no evidence to support the assumption that a nurse who is exceedingly sensitive to patient suffering is necessarily more effective in her nursing care. One might even argue that a certain degree of *in*sensitivity is psychologically necessary for a person who works for an extended period of time with patients who are undergoing extreme suffering. If a nurse sensitively and deeply empathizes with the suffering of every patient with whom he or she works, the psychological stress of his or her daily professional life might interfere seriously with the effectiveness of his or her functioning. Without further empirical evidence, however, these kinds of speculations must remain at an abstract level that provides little guidance either for nursing education or practice. This research, therefore, was designed to provide empirical evidence relevant to the clarification of this issue.

On the basis of these speculations, the following propositions were formulated as general guidelines for research:

1. *The suffering of another person is necessarily inferred rather than directly observed.* Thus, a nurse's judgment of the degree of suffering ex-

perienced by a patient depends upon a process of inference, though presumably the inference stems, in part, from the nurse's observations of the patient.

2. *An inference made from observations requires a cognitive process that either explicitly or implicitly takes the following general form: observation of cues; interpretation of these cues in terms of the experience of suffering; judgment of the other person's suffering.* The interpretation of cues involves an assignment of meaning to various cues in terms of the degree and nature of suffering. Thus, for example, for a particular nurse, one cue may mean high physical pain; another cue may mean high psychological distress. The interpretation of cues, therefore, depends upon the nurse's system of beliefs about the experience of suffering associated with various cues. In general, then, a nurse's reaction to a patient's experience of suffering is a function of observable cues and the nurse's belief system about suffering. Potentially relevant, observable cues include both verbal and nonverbal behavior of the patient, physical signs, nature of the patient's illness or injury, and characteristics of the patient such as age, sex, socioeconomic status, and ethnic background. The general concept of suffering may be thought of in terms of two basic dimensions: physical pain or discomfort and psychological distress.

The nurse's belief system may be viewed as a matrix of implicit assumptions relating observable cues to degrees of inferred physical pain and psychological distress. For example, one assumption in this belief system might be: Children suffer less pain than do adults. In this research, the set of implicit assumptions will be referred to as a *matrix of beliefs* or a *belief matrix*. The substantive nature of a belief matrix is defined by assumed relationships between specific observable cues and the degree of physical pain or discomfort and psychological distress a patient is experiencing. The belief matrix is a product of learning. Therefore, the substantive nature of a nurse's belief matrix is related to characteristics of the nurse likely to be associated with differences in patterns of social learning. Such characteristics include, for example, socioeconomic and ethnic background. There are individual differences among nurses in the substantive nature of their belief matrices, but because of common professional experiences, nurses also share certain commonalities. These commonalities are greater than those found among a group of randomly selected individuals in the general culture from which nurses come.

3. *In addition to their substantive nature, belief matrices may be distinguished from one another on the basis of the general level of inferred physical pain or discomfort and psychological distress.* This may be thought of in terms of a bipolar dimension. At one end of this dimension are nurses

who maximize the degree of suffering they infer in patients; at the other end are nurses who minimize their inferences of suffering. A nurse's relative position along the maximizing-minimizing dimension is a stable, enduring trait. Individual differences in the tendency to maximize or minimize patients' suffering are related to:

    a. constitutional factors (for example, nurse's pain threshold)
    b. life experience variables (for example, nurse's own experience with illness)
    c. social learning variables (for example, nurse's ethnic background)
    d. personality variables (for example, nurse's tendency to repress or attend to own psychological problems)
    e. professional experience variables (for example, nurse's area of specialization)

The tendency to maximize or minimize patients' suffering is also a function of certain relationship variables involving the patient and the nurse. These variables include, for example, the nurse's perceived similarity to the patient and the degree to which the nurse likes the patient.

    4. *Nurses' beliefs about suffering are related to their nursing behaviors in relation to patients.* In general, nurses who tend to infer relatively high degrees of suffering, in comparison to those who infer less suffering, are likely to be emotionally more supportive of the patient, more concerned with interpersonal and comforting aspects of nursing care, and psychologically closer to the patient as manifested in the emotional tone of communications and physical contact with the patient. In contrast, those nurses who infer relatively less patient suffering are likely to evince more interest in the technical aspects of nursing, to be less supportive of patients' complaints, and to be more distant both emotionally and in terms of their physical contact with patients.

    5. *The beliefs about suffering expressed by nursing students are likely to change over the course of their professional education.* These changes reflect both academic and clinical experiences concerned with patient suffering: (a) the acquisition of a professional role based on direct instruction as well as modeling; and (b) acculturation into the subculture of professional nursing. Although changes in beliefs are expected, at the outset of this research the specific direction of change could not be predicted.

Part Two

Nurses' Beliefs and Patient Characteristics

The first series of studies concerns nurses' beliefs about suffering in relation to certain patient characteristics. In these investigations our aim was to identify some of the relevant observable cues and to determine the relationships between these cues and reactions to both physical pain or discomfort and psychological distress. The specific variables considered in this series are: (1) socioeconomic status of the patient, (2) age of the patient, (3) ethnic background of the patient, and (4) nature of the patient's illness or injury.

2
Socioeconomic Status of the Patient

The first study in this series concerned the socioeconomic status of the patient. The research was designed to answer the following questions: Are nurses' reactions to suffering related to the patient's socioeconomic status? Did the fact that a patient was poor or wealthy, from an upper- or lower-class socioeconomic background, influence a nurse's judgment about the degree of physical pain or psychological distress the person was likely to experience? In addition to the variable of socioeconomic status, the research also investigated differences in reactions to suffering as a function of the nature of the illness, degree of severity, gender of the patient, and socioeconomic background of the nurse. In the analysis of results, each of these variables was considered singly as well as in interaction with each other. Thus, for example, the data provided a basis for determining whether or not nurses' judgments about suffering are related to the socioeconomic status of the patient, and if this relationship was a function of the nature of the illness, degree of severity, gender of the patient, or socioeconomic background of the nurse.

Method

Data were collected by means of a questionnaire asking nurses to rate the physical pain or discomfort and psychological distress of a series of patients. The variables of socioeconomic status of the patient, nature and severity of illness, and gender of the patient were manipulated by information provided in the questionnaire. The nurse's own socioeconomic background was evaluated on the basis of personal data provided by each subject (S).

Subjects

The Ss of this research were 50 female nurses, at the time of the study working in one of four large general hospitals in New York City, each with a staff of from 300 to 500 nurses. A description of the sample is presented in Table 2-1. As may be seen in this table, the nurses, on the average, had about nine years of experience, but the large standard deviation (7.28) indicates a fairly wide range of experience. A few of the nurses in the sample were recent graduates and some had been nurses for more than 20 years. In general, it seems reasonable to assume that, in terms of amount of experience, this sample is representative of the population of nurses currently working in large ci-

Table 2-1
Description of Subjects Who Participated in
Study Concerned with Socioeconomic Status of Patient

Number of Subjects	50
Years of Nursing Experience	
Mean	9.22
Standard Deviation	7.28
Current Position	
Staff Nurse	35
Head Nurse	1
Supervisor, Clinician	11
Director, Administrator, etc.	3
Areas of Nursing Experience	
General	35
Obstetrics, Gynecology	11
Pediatrics	4
Marital Status	
Single	31
Married	13
Divorced, Widowed	6
Socioeconomic Background	
Class 1	4
Class 2	6
Class 3	15
Class 4	8
Class 5	11
Class 6	4
Class 7	2
Country or Geographical Area of Origin	
United States and Canada	33
Orient	1
Europe	3
Caribbean	12
Africa	1

ty hospitals, and the results of this research can be generalized to nurses with varying degrees of professional experience.

The largest number of nurses in the sample were general staff nurses and a majority of the sample were unmarried. Socioeconomic background of the nurse was evaluated on the basis of the occupation of the major wage earner in the nurse's family during the period when she was growing up. Using Hamburger's revision of the Warner Scale (Hamburger, 1958), these occupations were rated on a seven-point scale, Class 1 representing what is usually considered high socioeconomic status (lawyers, physicians, engineers, and the like), and Class 7 representing the lowest status (migratory labor, messengers, and the like). As indicated in Table 2-1, the majority of nurses in this sample came from middle-class backgrounds (Class 3, 4, and 5), but the sample included the entire socioeconomic spectrum.

By and large, most of the nurses in this sample were born and raised in the United States and Canada, but a substantial minority (12) came from the Caribbean.

Instrument

Nurses' reactions to suffering were obtained by a 90-item questionnaire. Each item presented a brief vignette of a patient, with information about the patient's illness, gender, and socioeconomic status. The nurse was instructed to read the description of the patient and then indicate the degree of suffering she thought the patient was likely to be experiencing. For each item the nurse made two responses, first a rating of physical pain or discomfort on a seven-point scale running from *none* to *severe,* and then a rating of psychological distress on a similar seven-point scale.

Illnesses and injuries. Five categories of illness and injuries were included in the questionnaire: cardiovascular, trauma, psychiatric, cancer, and infection. These represent broad categories of illnesses encountered by nurses in general hospitals. Within each illness category, three degrees of severity were represented: mild, moderate, and severe. At this point in the research, our aim was not to establish rigorously quantitative definitions of severity. In a subsequent study reported in this series, results of an investigation specifically focused on the degree of suffering associated with a wide range of illnesses will be reported (see Chapter 5). However, for purposes of the present study, the goal was to identify three conditions within each illness category representing varying degrees of severity. To achieve these approximations, 63 nurses were asked to evaluate 69 illnesses and injuries as mild, moderate, or severe, and on the basis of these judgments, the three specific conditions within each category were chosen. A summary of the 15 conditions included in the questionnaire is presented in Table 2-2. Although not intended to be comprehensive, it seems reasonable to assume that these 15 illnesses and injuries approximate the range of conditions encountered by nurses within the five broad illness/injury categories.

Table 2-2
Illnesses and Injuries Used in Questionnaire Concerned with
Socioeconomic Status of Patient

Illness	Degree of Severity		
	Mild	Moderate	Severe
Cardiovascular	Low-grade systolic murmur	Thrombophlebitis	Aortic aneurysm
Trauma	Fractured arm several weeks ago	Fractured leg	Cervical Fracture (C4-5)
Psychiatric	Nervous, irritable	Debilitating anxiety	Psychotic behavior, reality loss, etc.
Cancer	Mole or lesion, pathology report negative	Possible leukemia	Leukemia confirmed
Infection	Abscess	Bronchopneumonia	Tetanus

Patients' socioeconomic status. The socioeconomic status of each patient described in a particular item was defined by occupation, as scaled by Hamburger's classification of occupations (1958). Each item in the questionnaire involved one of three categories of socioeconomic status (low, middle, or high) and a sample occupation such as hotel maid or watchman (low); lab technician, policeman or accountant (middle); banker, president of a large firm, or newspaper editor (high). In the vignette describing a particular patient, his or her occupation was mentioned in the course of the description. Thus, for example, an item involving a middle-class patient began with the sentence: "While demonstrating the features of a new model to a customer, Albert Warner, an automobile salesman, had what he termed a 'freak accident.' " Similar information about occupation was included in the vignette for each item.

Gender. Information about sex of the patient was conveyed by his or her name, care being taken to use names that were unequivocally associated with either males or females.

Instructions. The following instructions were given at the beginning of each questionnaire:

Each of the items in this booklet contains a brief description of a patient. Please read the description of each patient, and then judge the degree of physical pain or discomfort and the degree of psychological distress the patient is probably experiencing. Indicate your judgments about each patient by checking the appropriate places on the two rating scales for each item.

Remember, there are no right or wrong answers. We are only interested in your judgments. Do the ratings as quickly as you can. Don't sit and think for a long time about any one item. Read the description of each patient and quickly size up the case. Then, on the basis of your first reaction to the case, check off the two rating scales, indicating how much physical pain or discomfort and how much psychological distress you feel the patient is experiencing.

Ratings. Each rating was made on a seven-point scale, with the points on the scale defined verbally as follows: (1) none, (2) little, (3) mild, (4) moderate, (5) great, (6) severe, (7) very severe.

Note that, for the purposes of this research, neither physical pain nor psychological distress was defined for the subject. Such definitions were not included because the aim of this research was to explore the *nurse's own implicit beliefs* about suffering. An intrinsic part of this belief system is the nurse's own definition and understanding of physical pain and psychological distress. Therefore, definitions of these terms were omitted from any instructions given the nurse.

Format. Four variables were manipulated in the questionnaire: (1) illness, (2) degree of severity, (3) socioeconomic status of the patient, and (4) gender of the patient. A completely counterbalanced design was followed, such that each category of illness or injury was presented with each degree of severity, level of socioeconomic status, and gender. There were five categories of illness or injury, three degrees of severity, three levels of socioeconomic status, and two genders.

Illustrative of the items in the questionnaire is a vignette describing a male patient of high socioeconomic status with a cardiovascular illness of mild severity:

Kurt Oates, president of a large consulting firm, was feeling the effects of business pressures and thought he should have a physical checkup. A low grade systolic murmur was discovered and further diagnostic tests have been ordered.

Another item concerning a middle status, female patient with cancer defined as severe was as follows:

Running a steady fever of 103.6 and bleeding from the gums, chief dietician June Harris has been admitted to the hospital. Following a complete work-up, leukemia was conclusively diagnosed.

Personal Data

Prior to administration of the questionnaire, each nurse was asked to complete a personal data sheet. This included: (1) name, (2) years of nursing experience, (3) year R.N. license received, (4) current position, (5) area of most nursing experience, (6) marital status, (7) if married, spouse's job, (8) occupation of major wage earner in family when subject was growing up, (9) native country, and (10) ethnic or cultural background.

Nurse's socioeconomic background. Part of the personal data obtained from each nurse was the occupation of the major wage earner in the family when the nurse was growing up. This information was evaluated using Hamburger's occupational scale for rating socioeconomic class (Hamburger, 1958) and ratings of 1 to 7 were assigned. This rating provided a rough approximation of the nurse's social class background.

Consent forms. Before contacting a nurse in any of the participating hospitals, the general purpose and nature of the research was discussed with the director of nursing and other administrators in each hospital and a signed Institutional Consent Form was obtained.

At the first meeting with each nurse, before collecting any information, the research team provided subjects with information about the general nature of the study and offered to provide them with any feedback they desired when this phase of the research was completed. An individual consent form was obtained.

Procedure

For each of the four participating hospitals, the director of nursing asked for volunteers among members of the nursing staff. Data were collected during the nurses' regular work shift, and each hospital provided appropriate time off for the nurses to participate in the study.

A member of the research staff met subjects in each hospital in space provided by the hospital. On a randomly assigned basis, half the nurses were given Part One first (45 items) and half were given Part Two first (the other 45 items). Completion of either part required, on the average, between 30 and 40 minutes. Items were divided and sequenced in each part by random assignment.

Feedback to Subjects

Approximately three to four months after the data were collected, a member of the research staff met with small groups of subjects in the hospitals in which they worked to report and discuss the results of this research. In each instance, results obtained for the entire first series of studies were presented, and implications for both training and practice were discussed. These feedback sessions consistently generated a great deal of interest, enthusiasm, and discussion relating the research findings to the nurses' own experiences, and there were numerous requests to participate in further research along this line.

Analysis of Data

Ratings for physical pain or discomfort and psychological distress were treated separately, although the relationship between these ratings will be discussed in a subsequent study in this series dealing with nurses' views of suffering associated with various illnesses. Differences for each variable and their interactions were statistically evaluated by an analysis of variance using a repeated measures design. To achieve large enough subgroups for the analysis of nurses' own socioeconomic background, the 25 nurses in Classes 1, 2, and 3 were compared to those in Classes 4, 5, 6, and 7. Throughout the analysis of data, the null hypothesis was rejected at or beyond the .05 level.

Results

Physical Pain and Discomfort

The analysis of variance for ratings of physical pain showed that the differences in ratings of illnesses and degrees of severity were significant at the .001 level, and differences associated with the patient's socioeconomic status were significant at the .01 level. Neither the analysis for nurse's own socioeconomic background nor for gender of patient revealed statistically significant differences. All of the interactions were significant, most of them at or beyond the .01 level.

Interactions with Patient Socioeconomic Status

Table 2-3 presents the mean ratings of physical pain for each socioeconomic group of patients. The interaction between these variables was significant at the .001 level.

In general, low status patients were seen as suffering the greatest pain, with middle and high status patients approximately at the same level. This appears to be particularly evident with regards to both trauma and psychiatric illnesses. In contrast, for cardiovascular illnesses, low status patients were seen as suffering less than middle patients, who in turn were seen as suffering less than high status patients. The ratings by degree of severity and patient socioeconomic status indicate that nurses see a greater difference in physical pain between mild and severe illnesses for low status patients than they do for

Table 2-3
Mean Ratings for Each Illness
by Patient Socioeconomic Status ($N = 50$)

Illness	Socioeconomic Status			Total
	Low	Middle	High	
Cardiovascular				
physical pain	3.32	3.37	3.42	3.37
psychological distress	4.60	4.64	4.77	4.67
Trauma				
physical pain	4.55	4.26	4.24	4.35
psychological distress	4.64	4.50	4.65	4.60
Psychiatric				
physical pain	1.77	1.59	1.63	1.66
psychological distress	5.80	5.86	5.90	5.85
Cancer				
physical pain	3.05	3.00	3.13	3.06
psychological distress	4.65	4.91	4.75	4.77
Infection				
physical pain	4.34	4.34	4.29	4.32
psychological distress	4.39	4.22	4.25	4.29
Total				
physical pain	3.41	3.31	3.34	3.35
psychological distress	4.82	4.83	4.86	4.84

patients in the other two groups. Specifically, low status patients are believed to suffer less than others when the illness or injury is mild, but they are believed to suffer *more* when the condition is moderate or severe.

Although gender of the patient as a single variable was not related to amount of pain inferred by the nurse, there was a significant interaction between gender and socioeconomic status. Nurses see low status women as suffering *more* than low status men do, but high status women as suffering *less* than the parallel group of men.

Additional analysis. The main focus of this study was the patient's socioeconomic status, considered both as a main effect and in interaction with illness, severity, and gender. The data, however, permitted an examination of other interactions. There was a significant interaction between illness and degree of severity ($p \leq .001$), while the ratings for cardiovascular illnesses showed the greatest increase in perceived pain from the mild to severe categories. The mild cardiovascular illness was associated with little or no pain or discomfort, while the severe cardiovascular condition was seen as being considerably painful. In general, each illness category showed a somewhat different pattern of ratings along the dimension of severity. Inferences of pain for psychiatric illness fluctuated. Moderate psychiatric illness was perceived as less painful than either mild or severe illnesses of a psychiatric nature. Cancer showed an increase in perceived pain from mild to moderate and severe categories but not as large an increase as did cardiovascular illness. The sample of illnesses within each classification was too small to warrant generalizaiton. A fuller discussion of suffering associated with various illnesses will be presented in a subsequent study.

The illness-by-gender interaction was also found to be statistically significant, with males perceived as suffering more pain than females for cardiovascular illness, with the reverse true for infections.

Psychological Distress

The analysis of variance for ratings of psychological distress showed differences for illnesses and severity were significant at the .001 level. However, in contrast to the findings for physical pain, patient socioeconomic status in and of itself was not consistently related to the nurses' perceptions of psychological suffering. Nevertheless, all of the interactions involving the patient socioeconomic variable were significant (patient socioeconomic status-by-illness;-by-severity;-by-gender). Paralleling the findings for physical pain, the nurses' own socio-economic backgrounds were independent of their ratings of psychological distress.

Interactions with Patient Socioeconomic Status

The results summarized in Table 2-3 indicated that nurses viewed cardiovascular patients with high socioeconomic status as suffering psychologically more than others. Low status patients were seen as suffering somewhat *less* than others in cases of cancer and psychiatric illness, and somewhat more when the illness involved infection.

For severity of illness low status patients were seen as suffering least, in comparison to the other two groups, when the illness was mild or severe. The differences were small, though the interaction between these variables was statistically significant.

There was very little difference in the average ratings for male and female patients in either the low or high status groups, but there was a greater difference for the middle status group, with males seen as suffering greater psychological distress than females.

Additional analysis. The interaction between illness and severity was significant with marked differences in the patterns of ratings among the illness categories. For example, in the cancer category, there was relatively little psychological distress associated with the mild level of severity, undoubtedly reflecting the fact that the pathology report for these patients was reported to be negative. But there was a sharp increase in the ratings for those patients with a "possible" diagnosis of leukemia (moderate severity), almost as high as the rating for patients with a confirmed diagnosis of leukemia (severe). In contrast, patients with even a mild cardiovascular illness were seen to be experiencing considerable psychological distress, with somewhat smaller increases for the moderate and severe levels within this illness category. Infection showed a large increase in perceived psychological distress from the moderate to severe category while there was a larger increase in perceived distress for trauma from the mild to moderate category, with only a slight increase from moderate to severe trauma. There seemed to be a steady increase in the amount of psychological distress inferred from mild to moderate and severe psychiatric illnesses.

The gender-by-gender interaction was also significant, with males seen as suffering more under mild and severe conditions, and females suffering more when the illness is of moderate severity.

Summary of Findings for Socioeconomic
Status of Patient

1. Nurses' inferences of physical pain are consistently related to socioeconomic status of the patient, with low status patients generally seen to suffer more pain than either middle or high status patients.

2. Nurses' inferences of psychological distress are not consistently related to socioeconomic status of the patient. However, differences in amount of psychological distress associated with gender of the patient, nature of the illness, and degree of severity are indeed a function of the patient's socioeconomic status. Thus, while the socioeconomic variable in and of itself is a major determinant of nurses' inferences of physical pain, its effect on judgments of psychological distress is conditioned by other variables, such as patient gender and nature of the illness.

3. In view of the consistently significant interaction effects obtained for both physical pain and psychological distress, it is apparent that nurses' belief systems regarding patient suffering involve a complex matrix of variables. For example, while a patient's socioeconomic status influences nurses' judgments about physical pain, these judgments are also conditioned by other variables such as gender and illness. Similarly, a patient's socioeconomic status in interaction with other patient and illness characteristics influences nurses' judgments about psychological distress. In general, then, it seems reasonable to conclude that the socioeconomic

variable is an important one in nurses' belief systems about suffering, but it represents only one part of a matrix of variables that must be taken into account in understanding inferences of both pain and psychological distress.

4. The nature of the patient's illness accounts for a large part of the variance in nurses' inferences of suffering. This is true for both physical pain and psychological distress. Illustrating this proposition are the results obtained for cardiovascular illnesses: high status cardiovascular patients are perceived to suffer more physically and psychologically than lower status patients—a finding that runs counter to the general results, at least those for physical pain ratings.

5. Gender of the patient does not directly influence nurses' inferences of suffering. Nevertheless, gender does play a part in these inferences as a function of socioeconomic status. For example, in their inferences of physical pain, low status females are seen as suffering more than low status males, while the opposite is true for high status patients. Once again, the complexity of nurses' belief systems about suffering is underscored by these interaction effects involving gender.

6. Socioeconomic background of the nurse is not consistently related to inferences of suffering. However, this conclusion is tempered by the relatively restricted distribution of socioeconomic backgrounds among nurses in the sample. By and large, the majority of nurses in the sample came from families that are usually classified as middle and lower-middle class. There were relatively few nurses at either end of the distribution. Therefore, comparisons of nurses on the basis of their own socioeconomic background involved groups that were actually quite similar to each other along this dimension, and the null results for this variable may be accounted for by this restricted distribution.

3

Age of the Patient

The second study in this series posed the following question: Are nurses' inferences of suffering related to the patient's age? That is, did the fact that a patient was a child, young adult, or elderly person make a difference in nurses' inferences about the degree of physical pain and psychological distress the person was likely to experience? The data of this study also provided an opportunity to examine the effects of illness, degree of severity, and patient gender on nurses' beliefs about suffering.

Method

By and large, the methods of this research closely paralleled those described for the study of socioeconomic status. Therefore, descriptions of the instrument, procedure, etc. will be abbreviated, emphasizing only those aspects of the method which differed from the previously reported study. For those aspects of the method which are not specifically described in this section, it may be assumed that exactly the same procedure was followed as that reported for the study of socioeconomic status.

Subjects

The Ss of this research were 65 female nurses, at the time of the study on the staff of one of four large general hospitals in New York City. The nurses in this sample, like those in the study of socioeconomic status, had a wide range of experience. There was an average of over 7 years experience in nursing. Over half were staff nurses, and a substantial minority were currently in the position of head nurse (32 %). For the most part they characterized their area of practice as "General Nursing," rather than one of the more specialized areas of nursing. Nearly half of the sample was married, their socioeconomic backgrounds were primarily middle and lower-middle class, and the great majority were natives of the United States or Canada.

Instrument

Paralleling the instrument used to investigate socioeconomic status, the questionnaire developed for this study followed a complete counterbalanced design involving four variables: (1) illness, (2) severity, (3) age, and (4) gender. Thus, each illness was paired with each degree of severity, age, and gender. Given five categories of illness, three degrees of severity, four age groups, and two genders, a total of 120 items was required.

In the vignette for each item, the age of the patient was specified, representing one of the four age groups: children (ages 4–12); late adolescents and young adults (17–25); older adults (30–45); and elderly persons (over 65).

Illustrative of the items in the questionnaire is the following patient vignette involving a 17-year-old male with a cardiovascular illness of moderate severity:

> Mark Harrington, seventeen years of age, a member of the school's track team, felt discomfort in his left leg. An examination and further tests revealed thrombophlebitis which required hospitalization. Bedrest and anticoagulant therapy have been ordered.

Another representative item involved a 72-year-old male with an infection of mild severity:

> While pruning a hedge near his daughter's home, Edward Dennis injured his hand. At the insistence of his daughter, he finally saw a doctor. An incision and drainage of the abscess was performed in the office, and the 72-year-old man was told to soak his hand and return in three days.

For each item, the nurse was asked to rate on a seven-point scale the amount of physical pain or discomfort and the amount of psychological distress the patient was likely to be experiencing.

Analysis of Data

An analysis of variance with a repeated measures design was used to evaluate the results statistically.

Results

Physical Pain

The analysis of variance for ratings of physical pain showed the illness and severity variables to be significant beyond the .001 level of probability. Gender was significant beyond .05. The results for age, however, as a main

Table 3-1
Mean Ratings for Each Age Group by Patient Illness (N-65)

Age Group	Cardio-vascular	Trauma	Illness Psychi-atric	Cancer	Infection
4–12					
physical pain	3.34	4.24	1.98	3.09	4.05
psychological distress	4.47	4.68	5.64	4.00	4.46
17–25					
physical pain	3.30	4.33	2.12	3.06	4.03
psychological distress	4.72	4.89	5.87	4.95	4.30
30–45					
physical pain	3.38	4.29	2.01	2.78	4.06
psychological distress	4.92	4.77	5.72	4.92	4.52
65+					
physical pain	3.28	4.35	2.04	2.91	4.07
psychological distress	4.77	4.88	5.93	4.68	4.41

effect were not significant. All interactions were significant at the .01 level or above (most were at the .001 level), except the gender-by-age interaction which showed no statistically significant differences.

Age by illness. As indicated in Table 3-1, the same general pattern of pain ratings across illnesses was found for all age groups. Physical pain associated with psychiatric illness was rated lowest, while pain associated with trauma was rated highest. In between, cancer, then cardiovascular illnesses, and infections were rated in increasing order of pain. The significant interaction between age and illness was accounted for by differences between the amount of pain for one illness category and another; however, too few conditions were sampled in each category to warrant generalization about each category.

Psychological Distress

In contrast to the results obtained for ratings of physical pain, nurses believe that patients of various ages suffer different degrees of psychological distress ($p \leq .001$). The analysis of variance shows type of illness, severity of illness, and age all to be significant as main effects at the .001 level. Gender is significant at the .05 level of probability. All interactions are significant at .01 or beyond. Ratings of psychological distress for the three older groups (17–25, 30–45, and 65+) are remarkably similar (all within .04 of each other), but the mean rating for children (ages 4–12) is clearly lower than that of all other patients. Thus, while age and nurses' inference of physical pain are independent, nurses see children as suffering less psychological distress than any other age group of patients.

Age by illness. In addition to the significant main effect obtained for age, there is also a significant interaction between age and illness ($p \leq .001$). As shown in Table 3-1, the psychological distress experienced by both adolescents and young adults (17–25) and elderly persons (65+) in psychiatric illnesses is seen to be especially high. In contrast, the psychological distress of the 30–45-year-old group is viewed as particularly high for cardiovascular diseases. These findings are probably related to the incidence of various illnesses among the several age groups. The psychological distress associated with cancer is seen as relatively high for both the 17–25 and 30–45 age groups, somewhat lower for older patients, and much lower for children.

Age by degree of severity and gender. The interaction of age and severity is also significant ($p \leq .001$). The smallest differences in psychological distress among varying degrees of severity are seen for children and elderly persons, while the greatest differences are associated with the 17–25 and 30–45 groups. In this respect, nurses tend to see young and older patients in somewhat the same way. The significant interaction found for age and gender is reflected by the relatively small differences between males and females for both children and elderly persons and the much larger differences for the 17–25 and 30–45 groups. Thus, the findings for the age-by-gender interaction parallel those for the age-by-severity data in that both sets of results show a similar pattern for children and elderly persons in contrast to the other age groups.

Additional analysis. The results obtained for the interaction of illness by severity are essentially the same as those found in the parallel analysis in the study of socioeconomic status. By far the greatest difference in psychological distress occurs in the cancer category comparing mild severity (mole or lesion with negative pathology report) to a condition of moderate severity (possible leukemia). Similarly, as in the previously discussed study, the amount of psychological distress associated with a confirmed diagnosis of leukemia (a severe condition) is not a great deal higher than that seen for a possible diagnosis (a moderate condition).

In comparison to the other physical illnesses, even a mild cardiovascular condition is seen as involving a good deal of psychological distress, while the rating for infectious diseases remains low until the condition is severe.

For the illness-by-gender interaction, relatively small differences between male and female patients are seen for the four categories of physical illness, but for psychiatric illnesses, female patients are believed to suffer considerably more than males.

Summary of Findings for Age of the Patient

1. Age of the patient appears to have little influence on nurses' inferences of physical pain. However, age does play an important role in nurses' inferences of psychological distress.

2. Nurses believe that children, ages 4–12, experience considerably less psychological distress than patients in any other older age group.

3. Although children in general are seen as less distressed psychologically than other age groups, nurses' perceptions of other age groups are influenced by the nature of the illness. Thus, the psychological distress experienced by the 17–25 and 65+ groups with psychiatric illnesses is seen as especially high, while 30–45-year-old patients are believed to experience particularly high distress in cases of cardiovascular disease.

4. In studying the interaction of age with both severity and gender, it was found that nurses tend to see children and the elderly in similar ways in comparison to the 17–25 and 30–45-year-old groups.

5. As in the study of socioeconomic status, a large part of the variance in ratings of psychological distress is accounted for by the nature and severity of the illness. Each illness category shows a specific pattern of distress for the three levels of severity. For example, with the cancer category, there is little distress associated with the mild category, but nearly as much distress for the moderate degree of illness (a possible diagnosis) as there is for the severe degree (a confirmed diagnosis). In contrast, the amount of psychological distress inferred for a mild cardiovascular disease is relatively high, while the distress associated with infectious diseases is not seen as very great until the illness is severe.

4
Ethnic Background of the Patient

The third study considered the question: Are nurses' inferences of suffering related to the ethnic background of patients? To investigate this question, three sub-studies were conducted, each concerned with illnesses on one level of severity. This tri-part design was followed because a counterbalanced instrument involving all categories of ethnic background, illness, gender, and degrees of severity would have required administration of a large number of items (180) to each nurse. This would have required a great deal of time for each nurse, and the time available was necessarily limited. Therefore, for practical purposes, three parallel investigations were carried out, and the results are reported separately for each level of severity.

Illnesses of Mild Severity

Method

The same general method followed for the two studies previously presented was also followed in studying the effects of patients' ethnic backgrounds.

Instrument. As shown in Table 4-1, six categories of ethnic background were included in this research. There were: Oriental, Mediterranean, Black, Spanish, Anglo-Saxon/Germanic, and Jewish. Given five categories of illness and two genders, a total of 60 items was required.

Illustrative of the items in this questionnaire is the following vignette describing a Jewish female patient with a mild psychiatric condition:

Table 4-1
Variables Included in Questionnaires Concerned with
Ethnic Background of Patients

Illness	Ethnic Background	Gender
Cardiovascular	Oriental	Male
Trauma	Mediterranean	Female
Psychiatric	Black	
Cancer	Spanish	
Inflection	Anglo-Saxon/Germanic	
	Jewish	

Name: Sara Ginsburg
Age: 37
Background: Jewish
Symptoms: Nervous tension and irritability. Because of increasing irritability over minor events and a feeling that she was continually "ready to fly off the handle," Sara Ginsburg made an appointment to see a doctor. According to her, she was upset about many small things and felt edgy and sensitive.

The illnesses used in this questionnaire are listed in Table 4-1. All patients were identified as adults and their ethnic background was specified.

Subjects. The Ss of this study were 40 nurses, at the time of the study employed in one of four large general hospitals in New York City. About half of the sample were staff nurses, and a substantial minority were head nurses. Of the total sample of 40, 26 identified themselves as "General Nurses," while 9 were in obstetrics and gynecology, and 5 in other specialties. A majority of the sample were single, came from middle and lower-middle class backgrounds, and were born in the United States or Canada. Half the sample described themselves as Oriental, Mediterranean, Black, Jewish, or "other." The other half described themselves as Anglo-Saxon/Germanic. For purposes of statistical analysis, results for the Anglo-Saxon/Germanic group were compared to those obtained for nurses in all other categories of ethnic background.

Results

Physical pain. The analysis of variance indicates that illness was significant as a main effect at .001 and the ethnic background of the patient at .01. Differences in gender were significant at .05. Nurses' own ethnic background was independent of their ratings of physical pain. Illness-by-gender and illness-by-ethnic background of the patient were significant interactions ($p \leq$ .001) but gender-by-ethnic background of the patient was not significant at the .05 level or above. The mean ratings in Table 4-2 show that for mild ill-nesses, the nurses in this sample believe that Oriental and Anglo-Saxon/Germanic patients suffer least pain, while Jewish patiens suffer most, with Spanish patients second. There was no significant difference between the ratings of Anglo-Saxon/Germanic nurses and those from other ethnic backgrounds.

Our results suggest that ratings for Oriental patients are especially low for trauma and cardiovascular diseases, while Anglo-Saxon/Germanic pa-tients are seen as experiencing relatively little pain particularly when a psychiatric illness is involved. Jewish patients are generally seen as suffering more pain than others, and this seems to be most clearly evident for car-diovascular and psychiatric illnesses.

Psychological distress. The analysis of variance reveals that ethnic background of the patient and illness were statistically significant ($p \leq .001$). Patient gender was significant beyond the .05 level of probability but the nurses' own ethnic background was independent of their ratings of

Table 4-2
Mean Ratings for Each Ethnic Group of Patients
by Severity of Illness

| | Severity of Illness | | |
Ethnic Background	Mild (N-40)	Moderate (N-44)	Severe (N-48)
Oriental			
physical pain	2.24	3.43	3.90
psychological distress	3.15	4.80	5.65
Mediterranean			
physical pain	2.28	3.49	4.15
psychological distress	3.46	5.02	5.82
Black			
physical pain	2.24	3.52	4.09
psychological distress	3.20	4.90	5.67
Spanish			
physical pain	2.32	3.60	3.99
psychological distress	3.56	5.10	5.69
Anglo-Saxon/Germanic			
physical pain	2.27	3.48	3.94
psychological distress	3.13	4.97	5.51
Jewish			
physical pain	2.42	3.76	3.99
psychological distress	3.61	5.16	5.83

psychological distress. The illness-by-ethnic background interaction was significant ($p \leq .001$). The illness-by-gender and gender-by-ethnic background of patient interactions were not significant at .05 or above. Essentially the same pattern of results obtained for physical pain was also obtained for psychological distress. That is, Jewish patients were clearly seen as suffering the greatest psychological distress, with Spanish patients next, while Anglo-Saxon/Germanic and Oriental patients were seen as experiencing the least distress (Table 4-2).

With inferences of psychological distress relevant to the illness-by-ethnic background interaction, as in the ratings of physical pain (Table 4-3), Jewish patients were believed to be experiencing relatively high psychological distress under conditions of both cardiovascular and psychiatric illnesses, while the ratings for Oriental and Anglo-Saxon/Germanic patients were especially low for trauma and infections.

Illnesses of Moderate Severity

Method

Subjects. Forty-four nurses employed in the same hospitals as those described in the preceding studies participated in this research. These nurses had an average of over 7.5 years of nursing experience that encompassed a wide range of experience. Over two-thirds were staff nurses; almost 20 per cent were head nurses. The majority described themselves as working in the area of general nursing experience. A majority of these nurses were unmarried, came from middle-class backgrounds, and were originally from the United States or Canada. Half were of Anglo-Saxon/Germanic descent.

Instrument. The questionnaire used in this research was essentially the same as that described for the study of mild illnesses. The illnesses used in this study were those categorized in the moderate level of severity (see Table 2-2).

Results

Physical pain. The results for moderate illnesses essentially parallel those obtained for illnesses of mild severity. There was significant difference among ethnic groups ($p \leq .001$) and a significant illness-by-ethnic background interaction ($p \leq .01$). In addition, illness was significant as a main effect ($p \leq .001$) but gender of the patient and the nurses' own ethnic background were not. All other interactions were not significant. As shown in Table 4-2, Jewish patients were seen as suffering the most physical pain, with Spanish patients next, and Oriental patients seen as experiencing the

Table 4-3

Mean Ratings for Each Illness by Ethnic
Background of Patients

Ethnic Background	Cardiovascular			Trauma			Psychiatric			Cancer			Infection		
	Mild (N = 40)	Moderate (N = 44)	Severe (N = 48)	Mild	Moderate	Severe	Mild	Moderate	Severe	Mild	Moderate	Severe	Mild	Moderate	Severe
Oriental															
physical pain	1.04	3.78	4.04	2.61	4.50	4.96	2.07	2.35	1.96	1.90	2.82	3.46	3.22	3.67	5.10
psychological distress	3.54	4.40	5.19	2.46	4.86	5.69	4.42	5.54	6.45	2.46	5.06	5.95	2.85	4.17	5.00
Mediterranean															
physical pain	1.56	3.93	4.33	2.85	4.56	5.18	1.85	2.39	1.98	1.93	2.96	3.77	3.22	3.58	5.51
psychological distress	3.86	4.62	5.46	3.11	4.92	5.65	4.28	5.85	6.71	2.76	5.65	6.50	3.30	4.04	4.76
Black															
physical pain	1.42	3.75	4.18	2.60	4.87	5.26	2.02	2.44	2.18	1.96	2.98	3.38	3.20	3.69	5.46
psychological distress	3.59	4.36	5.11	2.69	4.62	5.35	4.40	5.92	6.74	2.32	5.32	6.12	3.48	4.27	5.02
Spanish															
physical pain	1.62	3.92	4.24	2.74	4.80	5.18	2.06	2.54	2.09	2.04	3.13	3.37	3.15	3.62	5.08
psychological distress	3.97	4.75	5.36	2.92	5.20	5.83	4.64	5.91	6.48	3.06	5.33	5.89	3.19	4.33	4.91
Anglo-Saxon/ Germanic															
physical pain	1.51	3.76	3.92	2.84	4.55	5.06	1.81	2.36	1.84	2.20	3.17	3.25	2.97	3.56	5.63
psychological distress	3.28	4.36	4.86	2.58	4.78	5.32	4.45	6.06	6.62	2.60	5.42	6.11	2.76	4.24	4.75
Jewish															
physical pain	1.67	4.26	4.22	2.81	4.77	4.97	2.13	2.85	1.83	2.28	3.15	3.50	3.23	3.74	5.38
psychological distress	3.95	4.82	5.55	3.06	4.92	5.55	4.79	6.15	6.87	3.10	5.46	6.12	3.12	4.45	5.06

least pain. Once again, the pain of Jewish patients was rated particularly high for cardiovascular and psychiatric illness (Table 4-3).

Psychological distress. The results were consistent with those previously reported. Significant differences were obtained for ethnic background ($p \leq$ .01) and for the illness-by-ethnic background interaction ($p \leq$ .001). Illness and gender were also significant as main effects but the nurse's own ethnic background was independent of her ratings of psychological distress for patients with illnesses of moderate severity. Two other interactions were significant: illness-by-gender ($p \leq$ .05) and gender-by-ethnic background of patient ($p \leq$ .01). As in the preceding study, nurses saw patients of various ethnic backgrounds as suffering different amounts of psychological distress, with Jewish and Spanish pateitns suffering most and Oriental patients least (Table 4-2). Once again, the psychological distress of Jewish patients, in comparison to others, was seen particularly under conditions of cardiovascular and psychiatric illnesses (Table 4-3). In contrast to the results for mild illnesses, ratings in this study showed a statistically significant interaction between gender and ethnic background. Oriental and black female patients were seen as suffering less psychological distress than their male counterparts, with little difference between sexes for the other ethnic groups.

Severe Illnesses

Method

Subjects. Forty-eight nurses participated in this study, and as a group they were very similar to the samples previously discussed. They had an average of over 10.5 years of nursing experience which included a wide range of experiences. The majority were general staff nurses who were single and from middle socioeconomic backgrounds. Most were originally from the United States or Canada. Half were of Anglo-Saxon/Germanic descent and over 20 percent were of black ethnic background.

Instrument. Using the illnesses listed as severe (Table 2-2, Chapter 2 p. 20), the same format was used as in the questionnaires for mild and moderate degrees of severity.

Results

Physical pain. Significant differences were obtained for ethnic background ($p \leq$ .001) and the illness-by-ethnic background interaction ($p \leq$ .001) The only other significant finding by the analysis of variance was illness as a main effect ($p \leq$ .001). Gender of the patient and the nurses' own ethnic background were independent of the ratings for physical pain. Illness-by-gender and gender-by-ethnic background were not statistically significant interactions. However, the pattern of ratings for this group was somewhat different. For severe illnesses, Mediterranean and Black patients were seen as suffering the most, and Oriental patients the least. The relatively high degree of suffering for Mediterranean patients was seen especially in cases of cancer and cardiovascular illness (Table 4-3).

Psychological distress. The analysis of variance showed that nurses believe patients of various ethnic backgrounds suffer different amounts of psychological distress ($p \leq .001$). Illness was also significant as a main effect ($p \leq .001$). Gender and the nurses's own ethnic background were not statistically significant. No interactions were significant. Jewish and Mediterranean patients were seen as suffering most, and Anglo-Saxon/Germanic patients least (Table 4-2).

Summary of Results for Studies of Ethnic Background

The results of the three studies dealing with the effect of patients' ethnic background on nurses' inferences of suffering were remarkably consistent. There were minor differences in the findings of the three studies, but in general, the following conclusions may be drawn.

1. Ethnic background of the patient was an important determinant of nurses' inferences of suffering. This was true for both physical pain and psychological distress.

2. In general, for both dimensions of suffering, nurses saw Jewish and Spanish patients as suffering most, and Oriental and Anglo-Saxon/Germanic patients as suffering least.

3. The most consistent and striking difference among ethnic groups involved nurses' perceptions of Jewish patients as suffering relatively greater pain and psychological distress in cases of psychiatric and cardiovascular illnesses.

5

Degree of Suffering Associated with Various Illnesses

Inspection of the analyses of variance reported for the preceding studies reveals that, in each case, a substantial part of the variance in ratings of suffering is accounted for by perceived differences among the various illnesses considered in the several questionnaires. Thus, it is apparent that the nature of a patient's illness strongly influences a nurse's inference of both physical pain or discomfort and psychological distress. In a sense, the nurse has certain expectations or beliefs about the degree of pain and psychological distress a patient with a given illness is likely to be experiencing, and these beliefs undoubtedly influence his or her judgments about the patient. To clarify further this aspect of nurses' belief systems about suffering, the present study investigated nurses' inferences of both physical pain or discomfort and psychological distress for a variety of illnesses encountered in hospital practice.

Method

The present research is a descriptive study designed to explore nurses' beliefs about the degree of suffering typically associated with various illnesses. The method of investigation, therefore, simply involved nurses' ratings of physical pain and psychological distress for a large number of illnesses and injuries.

Subjects

The Ss of this research were 81 nurses, at the time of the study employed in one of four large general hospitals in New York City. Like the samples previously described, the nurses in this study represented a wide range of experience in terms of the number of years of nursing experience. Most were general staff nurses, but there were a number of head nurses, and a variety of hospital nursing specialties (for example, obstetrics and gynecology, psychiatric, and pediatric) were included. The great majority were born in the United States or Canada, and in general, it seems reasonable to conclude that this sample was representative of nurses currently on the staffs of hospitals in New York.

Instrument

On the basis of consultation with a number of experienced nurses and nursing administrators, a list of 80 illnesses and injuries that nurses encounter in hospital practice was compiled. Obviously, such a list was not meant to be exhaustive; rather, the aim was to include a range of conditions, consistent with the experience of nurses in a large urban hospital.

Each illness or injury was listed, followed by two seven-point scales, one for a rating of physical pain or discomfort and the other for psychological distress. In contrast to the instruments used in the studies described in the previous sections, no information was given about the patient. For each item, the nurse was instructed to rate the amount of pain and distress that a typical patient with a particular illness or injury would probably experience.

Procedure

The same procedure for obtaining consent and ratings described in the reports of preceding studies was followed in this investigation.

Results

The rank ordering for mean ratings of physical pain or discomfort and of psychological distress for each illness or injury are presented in Table 5-1. A rank of *1* was assigned to the condition rated most painful (intractable angina) or involving the greatest psychological distress (cancer of the breast), and a rank of 80 was assigned to the condition rated least painful (low-grade systolic murmur) or least psychologically distressful (hematoma under thumbnail).

The average ratings covered a wide range along each dimension. Ratings of physical pain ran from a low of 2.29 (the scale-point of *2* was verbally designated as "Little Suffering") to a high of 5.61 (about half-way between the scale-points designated "Great" and "Severe"). The range for psychological distress was even larger, running from a low of 2.78 (just below the scale-point designated "Mild") to a high of 6.33 (nearly halfway between "Severe" and "Very Severe"). Thus, the aim of including illnesses and in-

Table 5-1
Ratings of Physical Pain or Discomfort and Psychological Distress for 80 Illnesses and Injuries (N = 80)

Illness	Ranking for Physical Pain, Discomfort	Ranking for Psychological Distress
Intractable angina	1	9
Second and third-degree burns of upper arm and chest; will require grafting	2	13
Second and third-degree burns anterior trunk and both legs; approximately 40 percent burn	3.5	17
Perforated duodenal ulcer	3.5	23
Broken neck	5	8
Gunshot wound of chest	6	30
Cholecystitis	7	65
Fracture at level of C(4–5) sustained in accident	8	18
Draining abcess of foot with cellulitis of leg and tender inguinal nodes	9	57
Pre-infarction angina	10	36
Rheumatoid arthritis	11.5	50.5
Meningitis	11.5	42
Stab wound of lower abdomen	13.5	38.5
Coronary thrombosis	13.5	34
Thrombosis of femoral artery with gangrene of foot	15	21
Draining abscess of foot with generalized septicemia	16	50.5
Chronic obstructive pulmonary disease	17	22
Fractured femur, sustained in accident	18	60
Coronary insufficiency	19	33
Hemorrhoids	20	74.5
Stab wound in arm	21	55
Bleeding from gums, temperature 103.6°F; diagnosis leukemia	22	1.5
Congestive heart failure with arteriosclerotic heart disease	23	41
Gunshot wound in leg	25	49
Thrombophlebitis	25	59
Bronchopneumonia in individual with chronic obstructive pulmonary disease	25	37
Hematoma under thumbnail	27	80
Abscess of hand requiring incision and draining	28	69
Bone tumor	29	20

Table 5–1 continued

Illness	Ranking for Physical Pain, Discomfort	Ranking for Psychological Distress
Nephritis	30	54
Nausea, vomiting, diarrhea	31.5	74.5
Upper respiratory infection; temperature of 104°F	31.5	67
Brain tumor	33	12
Hypertension, impending renal failure	34	27
Angina, relieved by nitroglycerine	35	46
Hodgkin's Disease	36	10.5
Leukemia	38	4
Thrombosis of femoral artery	38	52.5
Multiple Sclerosis	38	19
Four inch laceration of upper arm	40.5	66
Cancer of the bladder	40.5	10.5
Malignant hypertension	42	29
Arteriosclerotic heart disease, occasional dyspnea	43	48
Middle ear infection with symptoms of vertigo	44	64
Draining abscess of foot	45	77
Myasthenia Gravis	46.5	28
Undisplaced fracture of radius	46.5	72
Aneurysm, renal artery	48.5	42.5
Muscular Dystrophy	48.5	35
Varicosities of both legs	50	73
Prostatic cancer	51	15
Fractured clavicle sustained in an accident	52	78
Abdominal aortic aneurysm	53	44
Cancer of the breast	54	1.5
Concussion	55.5	70.5
Infectious Mononucleosis	55.5	70.5
Duodenal ulcer being treated with diet	57	63
Cancer of the uterus	58	7
Hepatitis	59	56
Hypertension	60	58
Tuberculosis	62	44.5
Epilepsy with grand mal seizures	62	47
Melanoma of thigh	62	30.5
Mitral Stenosis, preoperative mitral valve replacement	64	14

Table 5-1 continued

Illness	Ranking for Physical Pain, Discomfort	Ranking for Psychological Distress
Basal cell carcinoma of upper arm	65	32
Individual in panic state, eyes wide with terror; random, jerky movements	66	3
Feelings of anxiety accompanied with sweating, mild tremor of hands	67	16
Gonorrhea	68	68
General malaise, slight temperature, lethargy; being treated with fluids	69	79
Syphilis	70	61
Diabetes	71	62
Individual has feelings of anxiety and mild foreboding	72	38.5
Has difficulty sleeping, can't concentrate	73	52.5
Depressed and angry individual took three Sominex tablets; called hot line for help	74	5
Schizoid personality, goes to work, and is marginally productive	75	26
Feels sad and dejected, has some loss of appetite following death of a loved one	76	40
Progressive depression over many months; individual put affairs in order	77	24.5
Catatonic schizophrenia	78	24.5
Angry and suspicious, makes threatening gestures to everyone who approaches	79	6
Low-grade systolic murmur	80	76

juries that represented a broad range of both perceived physical pain and perceived psychological distress was achieved in the present instrument. Moreover, the standard deviations of ratings for all items was about one scale point, indicating fairly good agreement among the nurses in this sample about the degree of suffering "typically" experienced by a patient with each of the illnesses or injuries listed.

Over the 80 illness studied, the correlation between ratings of physical pain and psychological distress was 0.09, which of course was not significantly different from zero. Thus, across illnesses, nurses tended to see these two dimensions of suffering as independent of each other.

However, this conclusion must be qualified somewhat by the observation that, for some specific illnesses, nurses do see a relatively high congruence between amount of pain and amount of psychological distress. For example, nurses generally view severe traumas (for example second and third-degree burns, broken neck, fracture at level C (4–5)) as involving *both* a high degree of pain and psychological distress. Similarly, other relatively mild or clearly treatable conditions (diabetes, syphilis, general malaise, gonorrhea) are viewed as entailing relatively little pain and little psychological distress. An interesting minor side light of these findings concerns the relatively low psychological distress ratings for syphilis and gonorrhea. Both are in the lowest quartile of ratings for both dimensions of suffering. Twenty-five eyars ago, or perhaps in another setting today, these ratings for psychological distress would probably have been much higher. The present results undoubtedly reflect advances in treatment, changes in social mores, and perhaps the settings in which these nurses worked. Therefore, while the degree of pain and psychological distress are seen as independent when considered over the entire range of illnesses and injuries included in this study, there are conditions for which these two dimensions of suffering are seen as highly congruent with each other.

In general, nurses tended to infer a higher degree of psychological distress than physical pain for a given illness or injury. This was true for 62 of the 80 conditions considered; that is, the mean rating of psychological distress was higher than the mean rating of physical pain. Evaluating these results by a sign test indicates that this difference was statistically significant at the .001 level.

The conditions viewed as most painful tend to involve cardiovascular illness (for example, intractable angina, pre-infarction angina, coronary thrombosis, thrombosis of femoral artery with gangrene of foot) or severe trauma (for example, second and third-degree burns, broken neck, gunshot wound in chest, fracture at level of C (4–5), stab wound of lower abdomen). In addition, other specific conditions that do not fall into either of these two categories, such as a perforated duodenal ulcer and rheumatoid arthritis, were seen as especially painful.

In general, the conditions seen as least painful were those involving psychiatric illness, including even very severe psychotic conditions such as catatonic schizophrenia.

Among the conditions seen as psychologically most distressful, cancer was particularly evident. For example, of the ten conditions ranked highest in psychological distress, five involved cancer of one form or another. Other physical illnesses rated high for psychological distress included severe trauma (for example, broken neck) or severe cardiovascular illness (for example, intractable angina). Inspection of these results clearly suggested that physical conditions likely to result in death (cancer, severe cardiovascular illness) or extensive and long-term disability (for example, fracture at level C (4–5) were associated with high psychological distress. In addition, of course, severe psychiatric illnesses were seen as psychologically distressful.

Conditions seen as psychologically least distressful included a variety of minor illnesses and injuries, such as a hematoma under the thumbnail, a fractured clavicle, draining abscess of the foot, hemorrhoids, and infectious mononucleosis.

Summary of Findings for Degree of Suffering

1. In general, nurses tend to infer a greater degree of psychological distress than physical pain in evaluating the suffering typically associated with most illnesses and injuries.

2. Over a wide variety of illnesses, nurses' inferences of psychological distress are independent of their inferences of physical pain.

3. For some specific illnesses or injuries, however, nurses do see a high congruence between physical pain and psychological distress. This seems to be particularly true for severe traumas and severe cardiovascular illnesses; in these cases, a high degree of suffering is inferred along both dimensions. For other mild or clearly treatable conditions, little physical and psychological suffering is inferred.

4. Conditions viewed as physically most painful tend to involve severe trauma or cardiovascular illness, though specific conditions outside of these two broad categories are also seen as particularly painful.

5. In addition to various psychiatric illnesses, physical illnesses or injuries seen as psychologically very distressful typically involve the threat of death or long-term, severe disability.

Part Three

Individual and Group Differences Among Nurses

In this part several studies are reported dealing with individual and group differences among nurses in inferences of suffering. The first study describes the Standard Measure of Inferences of Suffering *used in most of the subsequently reported investigations. The next study deals with various correlates of individual differences among a group of American nurses, while the third chapter in this section reports cross-cultural differences among nurses from several countries. The fourth chapter deals with a comparison of black and white nurses in relation with black and white patients. The final chapter reports an exploratory investigation based on a study of highly empathic nurses.*

6

A Standard Measure
of Inferences of Suffering

In the several studies concerned with nurses' beliefs about suffering in relation to patient characteristics, the same basic strategy of measurement was used. A brief vignette describing a patient was presented and the nurse was asked to rate the degree of pain and psychological distress that a patient would be likely to experience. To investigate the effects of a particular patient characteristic such as age on nurses' inferences of suffering, the age of patients described in various vignettes was varied while other variables, such as nature of the illness or injury, were controlled. Thus, the variance in ratings accounted for by the particular characteristic under investigation could be determined.

The same basic design was followed in developing the *Standard Measure of Inferences of Suffering* (see Appendix, p. 191) to investigate individual and group differences among nurses. Five categories of illness/injury were used. These are: cardiovascular, cancer, infection, trauma, and psychiatric. Within each category two degrees of severity were considered: mild and moderate. Severe illnesses were excluded because of the relatively restricted range of ratings elicited by items involving more severe illnesses or injuries. The illnesses and injuries included in the instrument are the same as those in Table 2-2. However, only the mild and moderate conditions listed there were utilized in this study. Both male and female patients were described, and three age levels were used: 4–12, 30–45, and over 65. A counterbalanced design was followed, such that each illness/injury category was paired with each degree of severity, sex, and age level. There were five illness/injury categories, two sexes, and three age levels; thus, there were a total of 60 items.

Each item consisted of a brief vignette describing the patient's illness or injury, sex, and age. The subject was asked to make two ratings for each item: degree of physical pain and degree of psychological distress. Each of these ratings was made on a seven-point scale. Examples of the stimulus situations as included in this instrument are given in Figure 6-1.

Figure 6-1.

The Standard Measure of Inferences of Suffering Questionnaire*
(Selected examples of the total 60 items)

Tripping on an uneven pavement block, Louise Crane, 70 years old, fell and sustained a fractured femur. In traction at the moment, surgery is planned.

Physical pain, discomfort: 1 2 3 4 5 6 7

Psychological distress: 1 2 3 4 5 6 7

Concerned about the appearance of a mole on her upper left arm, 32-year-old Elizabeth Burdine decided to have the lesion removed in the doctor's office. The pathology report was negative.

Physical pain, discomfort: 1 2 3 4 5 6 7

Psychological distress: 1 2 3 4 5 6 7

36-year-old Gladys Lee stumbled and fell on the sidewalk, sustaining an abrasion of the hand. When the injury was not attended to, an abscess developed which required incision and drainage. She is to care for the hand through soaking and make an appointment to have the hand checked in a few days.

Physical pain, discomfort: 1 2 3 4 5 6 7

Psychological distress: 1 2 3 4 5 6 7

During a routine psychological test at his school, 7-year-old Austin Barett appeared troubled and concerned. When asked to arrange a series of blocks according to size and color, he insisted "they have sharp edges," and the "bright colors" bothered him.

Physical pain, discomfort: 1 2 3 4 5 6 7

Psychological distress: 1 2 3 4 5 6 7

Concerned about his difficulties standing on his feet for any period of time, 41-year-old Martin Downes was examined by his doctor. Thrombophlebitis was diagnosed. Currently he is in the hospital being treated with anticoagulant drugs while on complete bedrest.

Physical pain, discomfort: 1 2 3 4 5 6 7

Psychological distress: 1 2 3 4 5 6 7

---

*The complete Standard Measure of Inferences of Suffering Questionnaire appears in the Appendix on pages 191–202.

Reliability

The internal consistency of this instrument was evaluated on the basis of data obtained from 90 nurses. The average ratings of physical pain for even-numbered items was compared to parallel ratings for odd-numbered items. Using the Spearman-Brown correction, the correlation obtained was .96. For ratings of psychological distress, following the same procedure, a correlation of .96 was obtained. Thus, the instrument has a very high degree of internal consistency.

Test-retest reliability was evaluated by administering the instrument to 50 nurses on two occasions, one week apart. The test-retest correlation for ratings of physical pain was .89; for psychological distress .87. Therefore, this instrument was not only internally consistent, but also manifested a high degree of stability over time.

7

Correlates of Individual Differences in Nurses' Inferences of Suffering

Although our previous research has focused on central tendencies in inferences made by groups of nurses, all of the data thus far obtained reveal a considerable range of individual differences among nurses. Some nurses consistently infer a relatively high degree of suffering in patients, while other nurses consistently infer relatively little suffering. In this respect, the amount of suffering inferred by a nurse appears to be a stable characteristic of his or her belief system about suffering, and these beliefs differ from one nurse to another. The present research, therefore, was designed to investigate some possible correlates of these individual differences, with the aim of establishing an empirical basis for understanding why nurses differ in their inferences of physical pain and psychological distress.

Previous theory and research did not provide an adequate basis for formulating specific predictive hypotheses at the outset of this research. Nevertheless, observations of nurses, the folklore of nursing, and general psychological theory suggested a number of variables worth exploring.

For example, one might argue that, over the course of a nurse's career, as a result of repeated experiences with patients who have experienced suffering, a nurse might become inured to the pain and psychological distress of her patients. On the other hand, in the absence of systematic evidence, one might reasonably argue that nursing experience underscores the reality of patient suffering, and as a consequence, sensitizes the nurse to patient suffering. Without further evidence, it is difficult, if not impossible, to choose rationally one point of view or the other, but these considerations at least indicate that length of nursing experience is an important variable to investigate.

Similar reasoning led to the selection of a number of other variables. A nurse's position, for example, might influence his or her tendency to infer relatively high or low suffering. A nursing supervisor or head nurse often has more administrative responsibilities than a staff nurse, and as a result may have somewhat less patient contact, which in turn may influence his or her reactions to suffering. A nurse's area of specialization may also have some effect on sensitivity to patients' pain or psychological distress, with perhaps one area of nursing experience sensitizing the nurse to patients' pain while another area might lead to increased awareness of psychological distress.

National or ethnic background represents another variable worth exploring, but without evidence to warrant a specific prediction. It is commonly assumed that people from Anglo-Saxon/Germanic and Scandinavian backgrounds tend to be somewhat more stoic in their attitudes toward pain and psychological distress in comparison to those from Mediterranean and other cultural or ethnic backgrounds. This obviously reflects certain stereotyped beliefs about national, ethnic, or cultural differences, and such stereotypes often have little basis in fact. Nevertheless, national or ethnic background of the nurse seems worth considering in an initial exploratory study.

Along a somewhat different line, it seems reasonable to assume that a person's awareness of her own pain and psychological distress is related to that person's reactions to the suffering of others. For example, if an individual tends to experience a good deal of pain associated with her own illnesses and injuries, it might be reasonable to expect that person to infer a relatively high degree of pain among others who are ill or injured. Similarly, if a person is especially sensitive to her own psychological distress, that person may also be especially sensitive to the psychological distress of others.

Along a somewhat different line, Petrie (1967) has found that people consistently differ in the way they process various kinds of stimuli. For example, in a kinesthetic size judgment task Petrie found that some people tend to judge the size of an object as larger than it really is, others tend to judge it as smaller than it really is, and still others tend to be relatively accurate in their judgments. She classified these three groups as *augmenters, reducers,* and *moderates,* and in subsequent research found that augmenters have lower pain tolerance than do reducers or moderates. Thus, it would seem that augmenters judge the magnitude of pain stimuli as greater than do either reducers or moderates, just as they judge physical objects to be larger than do subjects in the other two groups.

Following Petrie's research, Vando (1969) began with the assumption that each individual strives to maintain an optimum level of stimulation, but some people "naturally" reduce stimuli while others augment stimuli. Therefore, a "reducer," in striving to achieve an optimum level of stimulation tends to seek stimulation to counteract his "natural" tendency to reduce the impact of stimuli. In contrast, an "augmenter" tends to avoid stimulation to counteract the natural tendency to increase the impact of stimuli. Vando developed a measure of the tendency to seek or avoid stimulation (*The Reducing-Augmenting Scale*) and found that people who preferred highly stimulating situations (reducers) had greater tolerance for pain, presumably because they reduced the impact of pain stimuli. In terms of the present research, it seemed reasonable to extend Vando's reasoning to the inference of suffering in others. That is, nurses who prefer highly stimulating situations might well be expected to reflect their tendency to decrease the impact of stimuli by inferring relatively less pain in others.

While the reducing-augmenting dimension presumably reflects perceptual processes that the individual may or may not be aware of, one might also expect conscious attitudes towards suffering to influence judgments about pain and psychological distress. A person who prizes stoicism, for example, might tend to infer relatively less suffering in others in comparison to those who do not have as strong stoic attitudes.

Finally, one might expect that a nurse's reactions to suffering would be related to the kind of nursing activities he or she prefers. Specifically, a nurse who is especially sensitive to psychological distress might focus on, and prefer, those aspects of nursing which emphasize the interpersonal relationship between the nurse and his or her patient or the patient's family. On the other hand, a nurse who was less sensitive to psychological distress might be more concerned with, and prefer, the more technical aspects of nursing.

In summary, the present research was designed as an exploratory study of some possible correlates of individual differences in nurses' inferences of suffering. To this end, measures of nurses' inferences of physical pain and psychological distress were obtained. These measures were studied in relation to the following variables: (1) years of nursing experience, (2) current position, (3) area of greatest nursing experience, (4) national or ethnic background, (5) reducing-augmenting reactions to stimuli, (6) reports of own pain experiences, (7) reactions to psychological distress, (8) stoicism, and (9) preference for interpersonal versus technical duties.

Method

Subjects

The subjects (Ss) of this study were 94 nurses who, at the time of the study, worked in two large metropolitan hospitals. As indicated in Table 7-1, the sample covered a very wide range of professional experience, from 1 year to 46 years, with a mean of approximately 8 years. Nearly half the sample was composed of staff nurses, while the rest of the sample included a large number of head nurses and others in supervising positions. Almost two-thirds of the sample were general medical-surgical nurses, with a much smaller number in pediatrics, psychiatry, and other specialties. The great ma-

Table 7-1

Characteristics of Sample in Study of Individual Differences
in Nurses' Inferences of Suffering ($N = 94$)

Item	Number
Years of Nursing Experience	
Mean	8.01
Current Position	
Staff nurse	43
Head nurse	24
Supervisor or other administrative position	27
Area of Greatest Nursing Experience	
Medical–surgical	61
Pediatric	8
Psychiatric	13
Other	12
Country of Birth	
United States	86
Other	8
Ethnic or National Background	
North European	51
South European	14
East European	9
African	19
Oriental	1

jority were born in The United States, with over 50 coming from Northern European backgrounds, and the remainder representing other backgrounds.

Inference of Suffering

Three scores were obtained on the basis of each S's responses to the *Standard Measure of Inferences of Suffering*. These scores were: (1) mean pain rating, (2) mean psychological distress rating, (3) mean of pain plus psychological distress ratings. Each of these means, of course, was computed over the total of 60 items in the instrument.

Own Pain

A measure of each S's own experience of pain was obtained by a twenty-item questionnaire in which the S indicated the degree of pain or discomfort felt the last time he or she experienced each of a series of events commonly associated with some pain. For example, the first item asked the *S* to indicate the amount of pain or discomfort felt the last time a headache was experienced using a seven-point rating scale that ranged from (1) none, to (7) very severe. Other items asked for ratings of pain associated with experiences such as a sore throat, a stomach ache, a dentist drilling your tooth, an injection. The mean rating over the 20 items was computed, and a high score indicates a tendency to report a relatively high degree of pain.

Reducing-Augmenting Scale

The tendency to seek or avoid stimulation was measured by a 28-item forced choice scale. Each item presented two stimulus situations, one involving high stimulation and the other low stimulation, and the *S* was asked to choose the one she preferred. Thus, for example, an *S* was asked to indicate his or her choice of: (*a*) loud music, or (*b*) quiet music; (*a*) water skiing, or (*b*) boat rowing; (*a*) security, or (*b*) excitement. Vando (1969) developed this instrument and he reports a split-half reliability of 0.89 and a test-retest reliability of 0.74. A high score on this instrument indicated a preference for relatively high stimulus situations, theoretically reflecting a tendency to reduce stimulation.

Repression-Sensitization Scale

Sensitivity to one's own experiences of psychological distress was measured by the *Repression-Sensitization Scale* developed by Byrne (1961). This scale has been widely used in previous studies and has proven to be a reliable as well as useful instrument for measuring the degree to which a person pays attention to, and reports, feelings of psychological distress. The instrument was composed of 156 true-false items; a high score indicated sensitivity to one's own feelings of distress and a low score indicated a tendency to repress these feelings.

Preference for Interpersonal versus Technical Duties

To measure each *S*'s preference for interpersonally oriented versus more technical nursing duties, the *S* was asked to rank 12 nursing activities, from the one he or she was most interested in doing (ranked 1) to the one he or she was least interested in doing (ranked 12). Five of these activities involved interpersonally oriented activities, such as to provide reassurance and psychological support for an anxious patient. The other seven statements concerned more technical activities, such as irrigate ear, nose, or throat. The score obtained from this instrument was the average rank of the five interpersonally oriented statements. Thus, a small score reflected relatively high ranks for these statements, indicating high interest in interpersonally oriented activities, while a large score reflected relatively lower ranks, indicating higher interest in technically oriented activities.

Stoicism

The degree to which a person espoused stoic attitudes was measured by a 10-item scale. Each item consisted of a statement reflecting a general stoic attitude, and the *S* was asked to indicate agreement with the statement on a six-point scale running from strongly agree to strongly disagree. Representative statements reflecting a stoic attitude included: (a) In general, many people tend to complain too much, (b) When pain and discomfort are inevitable, the best thing to do is grin and bear it, (c) I admire people who can bear pain without complaining. The 10 statements used for this instrument were selected from a list of 30 statements on the basis of 50 judges' ratings of the degree to which each statement reflected a more general stoic attitude. Test-retest reliability obtained with 60 Ss over a two-week interval was .86. A low score on this instrument indicated a relatively high stoic attitude.

Procedure

Potential *S*s in each hospital were met in small groups of three to ten nurses. The general nature of the research was explained by a member of the project research staff and the nurses were asked to participate on a volunteer basis. Data analysis was based on the 94 *S*s who completed all of the measures involved in the research.

An attempt was made to collect data from each nurse in two sessions. This was not always possible because of work schedules. The instruments were administered in the following order: (1) identifying data questionnaire, (2) preference for interpersonal versus technical nursing activities, (3) the standard measure of inferences of suffering, (4) reports of own pain experiences, (5) reducing-augmenting scale, (6) repression-sensitization scale, and (7) stoicism scale. The average time required for data collection for each *S* was approximately two-and-one-half hours.

Statistical Analysis

For measures producing continuous scores, the data were analyzed by means of product moment correlations. Thus, correlations among the following variables were computed: years of experience, mean pain rating, mean psychological distress rating, mean of pain plus psychological distress ratings, reports of own pain experiences, reducing-augmenting, repression-sensitization, and stoicism. A chi-square analysis comparing nurses at the extremes of the inferred suffering measures was computed for the following variables: current position, area of greatest nursing experience, and national or ethnic background.

Results

Before analyzing the results for the entire sample of 94 nurses, the data for nurses working in the two hospitals were compared. There were no significant differences between these groups for any of the variables considered in the subsequent analysis. In fact, the two samples were, on the average, very similar to each other in all relevant dimensions. Therefore, the data for the two hospitals were pooled for the following analyses.

Table 7-2 presents the intercorrelation matrix. As indicated in Table 7-2, ratings of one's own pain and the tendency to augment stimulation are related to nurses' inferences of patients' physical pain. Thus, a nurse who tends to view patients as suffering relatively high physical pain also tends to report that he or she has suffered relatively high pain in his or her own experiences. In addition, the nurse who tends to infer relatively high pain also tends to augment stimulation. However, repression-sensitization, stoicism, and years of experience are independent of mean pain ratings.

Inferences of psychological distress are related to a preference for interpersonally oriented nursing activities. However, all of the other measures are independent of mean psychological distress ratings. When ratings of physical pain and psychological distress are combined, the pattern of correlations changes only slightly. Only ratings of own pain and the tendency to augment stimulation are significantly related to the combined measure of inferences of suffering.

In the analyses for current position, area of greatest experience, and ethnic or national background, for each variable the 24 nurses in the sample who had highest mean ratings of pain and psychological distress were compared with the 24 nurses who had the lowest ratings. For the analysis of current position, the supervisory and administrative categories were collapsed in order to achieve frequencies sufficient for a chi-square analysis. This analysis showed that there was virtually no difference between the upper and lower quartiles of the sample on mean ratings in terms of whether the nurses were staff nurses or not. Similarly, to achieve adequate frequencies for the analysis of areas of greatest nursing experience, categories other than medical–surgical nursing were collapsed. The chi-square analysis revealed no significant difference between the upper and lower quartiles on ratings for the area of experience variable.

For the analysis of ethnic or national background, the *Ss* were classified into three categories: North European, Other European (including East and South European), and African. The chi-square analysis revealed a statistically significant difference in the backgrounds of *Ss* in the upper and lower quartiles of the inference of suffering distribution. In the lower quartile (in other

Table 7-2
Correlations between Variables Considered in Study of
Individual Differences in Inferences of Suffering ($N = 94$)

	$\bar{X}$ Pain	$\bar{X}$ Psychological Distress	$\bar{X}$ Pain plus Psychological Distress	Own Pain	Reducing-Augmenting	Repression-Sensitization	Stoicism	Years Experience	Interpersonal-Technical Preference
$\bar{X}$ Pain		.56***	.86***	.32***	−.17*	.10	.07	−.14	.08
$\bar{X}$ Psychological distress			.90***	.15	.13	.09	.03	.11	−.17*
$\bar{X}$ Pain plus psychological distress				.26**	−.17*	.11	.06	.00	−.15
Own pain					.07	.27**	−.30**	.15	.09
Reducing-augmenting						.10	.11	−.22*	.09
Repression-sensitization							−.06	−.21*	.10
Stoicism								−.32**	−.23*
Years experience									.03
Interpersonal-technical perference									

*$p \leq .05$
*$p \leq .01$
***$p \leq .001$

words, those who inferred relatively low patient suffering), there was a clear predominance of nurses from North Eurpoean backgrounds. In the upper quartile, there were three times as many Ss from Other European as in the lower quartile, and twice as many from African backgrounds inferred relatively high patient suffering in comparison to low ratings.

Secondary analyses. Although the primary aim of this research concerned correlates of inferences of suffering, intercorrelations among the other variables were of some interest. These results indicated that those *S*s who had a relatively greater number of years of nursing experience (and were generally older) tended to prefer less stimulating situations, complained less of psychological distress, and professed more stoic attitudes. In general, those *S*s who reported their own experiences as relatively painful also tended to report more psychological distress and revealed less stoic attitudes. Finally, those who reported more stoic attitudes generally reported lower preference for interpersonally oriented nursing duties.

Discussion

Nurses who infer relatively greater patient pain tend to report their own experiences as more painful and also tend to augment the impact of a variety of stimuli. Nurses who infer relatively greater psychological distress show some tendency to prefer interpersonally oriented nursing duties. In general, nurses from Eastern and Southern European or African backgrounds tend to infer greater patient suffering than do nurses from Northern European backgrounds. However, repression-sensitization, stoic attitudes, years of experience, current position, and area of greatest nursing experience were unrelated to inferences of suffering.

The highest correlate of ratings of patient pain is ratings of one's own pain ($r = .32, p \le .001$). This observed relationship might be accounted for by a general response tendency to give relatively high ratings, regardless of the specific nature of what is rated. However, the fact that inferences of pain are *not* related to several of the other measures obtained mitigates against this interpretation. That is, if the relationship between inferences of other's pain and reports of one's own pain is merely a function of a response set, one would expect this set to be reflected in the other measures. This is not the case in the present data, and it therefore seems reasonable to interpret these results in terms other than as a consequence of a general response set. Specifically, these results suggest that nurses who experience greater pain themselves tend to infer greater pain in others. This finding is obviously congruent with the general point of view underlying this entire line of research, which began with the assumption that one person can never directly observe another person's suffering. Thus, "knowledge" of another person's suffering is always a matter of inference, and the inference depends upon one's own experiences and beliefs. A model of the inferential process might be formulated in terms of the following hypothetical syllogism:

> The other person is undergoing a particular illness or injury. If I were undergoing that particular illness or injury, I would probably be experiencing a certain degree of pain (based on one's own experiences and beliefs about pain). Therefore, I infer that the other person is experiencing approximately the same degree of pain that I would experience under a similar condition.

We are not suggesting that a nurse necessarily follows this formal model in her conscious thinking about a patient, but it does seem reasonable to assume that the inferential process follows this general model regardless of whether or not the nurse is aware of each step in her thinking.

In designing this research it was assumed that the *Repression-Sensitization Scale* would provide a self-oriented parallel to inferences of others' psychological distress, just as ratings of one's own pain paralleled inferences of others' pain. However, a post hoc examination of this scale suggests that this assumption may not have been warranted. The *Repression-Sensitization Scale* reflects the *number* of different psychological symptoms of distress a person reports, while the inference of a patient's psychological distress involves an estimate of the *intensity* of psychological suffering another person is experiencing. Thus, one measure deals with number of different symptoms of suffering and the other measure deals with intensity or degree of suffering. In future research, therefore, inferences of patients' psychological distress should be investigated in relation to a measure of the reported intensity of psychological distress experienced by the nurse herself in a variety of illness and injury conditions. Data obtained by these measures would provide a more appropriate test of the general hypothesis that inferences about another person's experiences are based, in part, on one's own experiences under similar conditions.

The only other correlations to reach a statistically significant level involved the Reducing-Augmenting Scale and the preference for interpersonal versus technical nursing duties. However, these correlations were so low ($r = -.17, p \leq .05$) that, in view of the number of correlations computed, one cannot conclude with confidence that these results can be generalized from the present sample. In any event, neither of these variables appears to account for much of the variance in inferences of suffering, and they do not seem to represent profitable lines for further investigation.

Much more promising are the results obtained for ethnic or national background. The findings of this study are congruent with the results of our earlier cross-cultural research, which revealed significant differences in inferences of suffering reported by nurses in various countries. The results of the present study indicate that, not only do nurses in various countries differ in their inferences of suffering, but nurses in the United States who have various national and ethnic backgrounds also differ in their inferences about patients. Thus, the nurse's cultural background is an important determinant of her beliefs about pain and psychological distress. On the basis of the present results, one would expect an American nurse whose background is African, South or East European (Italian, Spanish, Russian, Polish, and the like) to infer relatively high patient suffering. In contrast, an American nurse from a North European background (English, Irish, German, Scandinavian) would be more likely to infer relatively less suffering. There are undoubtedly many exceptions to these general propositions, but they do reflect general trends in the present data.

The findings suggest that belief systems about the suffering of others are influenced both by an individual's own experiences of suffering and socially learned attitudes about pain and psychological distress. Thus, a nurse who has experienced a great deal of pain associated with a particular injury may believe that another person with a similar injury is also experiencing a high level of pain. But this belief is also influenced by his or her attitudes toward pain, attitudes acquired as a consequence of his or her history of social learning. The results of this research demonstrate that a nurse's ethnic or cultural background is an important factor to consider in his or her history of social learning, but it would also be important to investigate in greater detail the social learning that occurs in the course of a nurse's training and professional experience. The findings of this study suggest that, after at least one year of professional practice, nurses' inferences of suffering do not change consistently. Years of experience relate to reducing-augmenting stimulation, repression-sensitization, and stoic attitudes, but not to inferences of suffering. Therefore, the important social learning that occurs in this regard may well occur during a nurse's training and early in professional practice. Further research designed to investigate changes in nurses' beliefs during training and early in practice is currently being planned, with the aim of further explicating the factors that influence a nurse's inferences of suffering.

8

Cross-Cultural Differences in Nurses' Inferences of Suffering[1]

The purpose of this study was to investigate possible cross-cultural differences in nurses' inferences of suffering. Our basic rationale stems from the assumption that the inference of suffering in others is a socially learned behavior. That is, within a given society, an individual learns from others the culturally appropriate interpretation and response to cues associated with suffering. In one society, for example, people may believe that a particular illness is commonly associated with great suffering; in another society, people may believe that the same illness involves moderate or minimal suffering. Thus the cultural system of beliefs about illness and suffering influences a nurse's inferences about the experiences of the patients with whom he or she works. It is further assumed that these belief systems of suffering are a function of a particular culture's values and customs. In one culture, for instance, stoicism and emotional control may be prized, and one might expect members of this culture to minimize the degree of suffering experienced by others. In another culture, emotional responsiveness may be prized, and members of this culture might be expected to maximize their inferences of suffering. Since cultures differ in customs, values, and ways of perceiving and interpreting various phenomena, one would expect nurses from various cultures to differ in their inferences of suffering associated with illness and injury.

The cultural belief system relevant to inferences of suffering is primarily concerned with the association of various illnesses or injuries and degree of suffering a patient is assumed to be experiencing. This belief system is likely to be influenced by other cultural values. A specific culture's characteristic attitude toward age, for instance, might influence beliefs about suffering. A

[1]This study was conducted in conjunction with Dr. Yasuko Sameshima Higuchi, and the authors wish to express their deep appreciation to Dr. Sameshima for her invaluable contributions to the research. We also wish to thank the American Nurses' Foundation for their encouragement and support of the various cross-cultural studies.

society that places special positive value on age, in contrast to a society that emphasizes youth, is probably characterized by different beliefs about the association of illness and suffering that are related to the age of the patient. In one society, the suffering of the aged may be emphasized. In another society, the suffering of children may be emphasized. One would therefore expect an interaction between age of the patient and cultural differences in degree of suffering inferred.

Following the same general line of reasoning, as a consequence of cultural differences in the perception of male and female roles, it is reasonable to predict an interaction between the sex of the patient and differences in inferred suffering.

Finally, cultures differ in beliefs about the relationship between body and mind, between the physical and psychological. In one culture, it is assumed that physical and psychological phenomena are intimately related, and that psychological events closely parallel physical events. In another culture, physical and psychological phenomena are assumed to reflect very different realms, and psychological events may be thought of as quite independent of physical events. One would therefore expect cultural differences in the relationship between inferred physical pain or discomfort and psychological distress.

Hypotheses

The specific hypotheses tested in this study are the following:

1. Degree of patient suffering inferred by nurses is related to national background of the nurse, such that nurses in the United States, Japan, Taiwan, Korea, Thailand, and Puerto Rico differ in the degree of suffering inferred from the same patient descriptions. This is true for inferences of both physical pain and psychological distress.

2. There is an interaction between both illness and its severity and national background in the degree of suffering inferred by nurses. That is, degree of suffering inferred about patients of different illnesses and severity is related to national background of nurses.

3. There is an interaction between age of patient and national background in the degree of suffering inferred by nurses. That is, degree of suffering inferred about patients of different ages is related to national background of nurses.

4. There is an interaction between sex of patient and national background in the degree of suffering inferred by nurses. That is, degree of suffering inferred about patients of different sexes is related to national background of the nurses.

Method

Subjects

Participants in this study consisted of a total of 544 female registered nurses at the time of the study employed in the United States, Japan, Puerto Rico, Korea, Thailand, and Taiwan. In general, groups of nurses in the several countries sampled were similar to each other along major relevant dimensions. The average age was almost 30 and the mean years of nursing experience was 7.61 which included a wide range of experience, 70 percent being staff nurses. Over half of the nurses in this sample were single, 63 percent were graduates of three-year training programs, and 20.4 percent were graduates of four- or five-year programs. However, some trends in these background characteristics might be noted. American nurses tended to be somewhat older than those in most other groups, and to have had more experience in nursing. Half were in staff positions; more than half were married. Less than half were diploma school graduates and one-third were graduates of A.D. programs. Japanese nurses tended to be older and more experienced in nursing than any other group; almost all were diploma school graduates. About half were staff nurses, and the other half were head nurses and administrators; more than half were single. Puerto Rican nurses were the third oldest group and were more experienced than Korean, Thai, and Taiwan nurses. A majority held staff positions and were married, and about half were diploma school graduates. Among the groups studied, Korean nurses were the youngest and had the least experience in nursing. Almost all were staff; a majority were single and graduates of diploma programs. Thai nurses were also relatively younger than the other groups and had less experience; a majority held staff positions, were single, and graduates of diploma programs. The nurses from Taiwan were also younger than American and Japanese nurses, and less experienced. The majority were staff nurses; more than half were single. Their educational background included A.D., diploma, baccalaureate, and graduate programs.

Instruments

The *Standard Measure of Inferences of Suffering* was used to obtain ratings from nurses in all of the countries involved. For testing in countries other than the United States, the instrument was translated into Japanese, Korean, Thai, Spanish, and Chinese. Translators were native speakers of the respective languages, and whenever possible, they were also registered nurses. To insure accuracy of translation, a back-translation method was used. For each language, the translated version of the questionnaire was independently translated by another native speaker into standard English. Other than difference in language, the only other substantive difference between the original English version and that in any other language was the substitution of appropriate common names for patients in their country.

Procedure

Data in the United States were collected by members of the research staff. In each of the other countries, one nurse in a major administrative position was contacted and served as the coordinator of data collection for the particular country involved. All except one of these coordinators had previously been students of one of the principal coinvestigators, thus providing a personal basis for this cooperative effort. The general purpose of the research was explained to the coordinators, who then supervised the data collection in their respective countries.

Results

The first hypothesis predicted that nurses in the several countries sampled would differ in the degree of suffering inferred. Table 8-1 presents the mean physical pain and psychological distress ratings for each national group. The analyses of variance clearly and strongly supported the first hypothesis that degree of patient suffering inferred was related to the national background of the nurse in terms of all the major variables considered in this study ($p \leq .001$).

The specific pattern of ratings in the several countries was not predicted, and thus firm conclusions about these patterns could not be drawn on the basis of the present results. Nevertheless, the data proposed some interesting considerations. In particular, the Korean and Japanese samples showed the highest inferences of physical pain, and nurses from the United States and Puerto Rico inferred the lowest degree of physical pain. The nurses from Taiwan tended to infer a moderate degree of physical pain with the smallest variability in ratings. The mean ratings of psychological distress

Table 8-1
Mean Ratings for Each Country

Country	Mean Rating of Physical Pain	Mean Rating of Psychological Distress
United States	3.00	4.43
Japan	3.73	4.64
Puerto Rico	3.06	4.80
Korea	3.81	4.84
Thailand	3.20	4.40
Taiwan	3.54	4.06

for all cultural groups were higher than for physical pain. The nurses from Korea and Puerto Rico inferred the greatest degrees of psychological distress, and the Taiwan sample inferred the least suffering of all the groups. The sample from the United States was in the middle of the other national groups, and the variability was smallest. In terms of the sum of both physical pain and psychological distress, Japanese and Korean nurses gave the highest mean ratings of all groups. The greatest differences between physical pain and psychological distress were among Puerto Rican nurses followed by American nurses. In contrast, the Taiwan sample showed the smallest difference between the two aspects of suffering considered in this research.

Interaction of Illness, Severity, and National Group

The analyses of variance of the ratings of physical pain and psychological distress in the study of five diseases (trauma, cancer, infection, cardiovascular, and psychiatric), two degrees of severity, and the six cultural areas supported the predicted hypothesis of an interaction between illness and severity of the illness in the patient and the cultural background of nurses. Differences among the six different national groups were statistically significant for both physical pain and psychological distress for five illness and two severity variables (most at $p \leq 0.001$).

The physical pain ratings for the five illness variables for each culture showed that the Korean and Japanese samples tended to infer greater pain than the other national groups. The Korean sample showed the highest ratings for trauma, cardiovascular, and psychiatric illnesses, and the Japanese sample showed the highest for cancer and infectious diseases. The United States and Puerto Rican samples tended to infer less pain than other groups. The sample from the United States showed the lowest inference in trauma, infections, and cardiovascular diseases, and the Puerto Rican sample showed the lowest ratings for cancer and psychiatric diseases. All cultural groups exhibited the same rank order of illness categories; the highest mean was trauma, followed by infections, cardiovascular, cancer, and psychiatric disease.

For psychological distress the Korean and Puerto Rican samples showed higher mean ratings than all other groups. The Korean sample showed the highest mean ratings in trauma and psychiatric illnesses and the Puerto Rican sample showed the highest mean ratings for cancer. The Japanese sample showed the highest mean ratings in infections and cardiovascular diseases. The Taiwan sample showed the lowest psychological distress in all disease categories. All cultural groups inferred the highest psychological distress for psychiatric illness.

For physical pain ratings of the two severity categories for each different national group, the Korean sample showed the highest rating in the mild illness category and the sample from the United States the lowest rating.

In the moderate illness category, the Japanese sample showed the highest and the Puerto Rican sample the lowest mean rating.

For psychological distress ratings of two severity categories for each national group, the Puerto Rican sample shows the highest mean rating in the mild category, while for the moderate category, the Japanese sample shows the highest mean. The Taiwan sample showed the lowest mean ratings of all groups for both mild and moderate categories.

Interaction of Age and National Group

The third hypothesis predicted an interaction between age of the patient and national group. The analyses of variance for physical pain and psychological distress within the three age groups showed statistically significant differences among the six cultural groups. For physical pain ratings the 4–12 age group versus the 35–45 age group interaction was significant (at $p \leq .01$). All other main effects and interactions were significant (at $p \leq .001$). The analysis for ratings of psychological distress revealed all age groups significant as main effects (at $p \leq .001$). All interactions of age groups were also significant at the .05 level or beyond. Thus, the third hypothesis, which predicted an interaction between age groups of patients and cultural background of nurses, was clearly supported.

A summary of the mean ratings for the three age groups (4–12, 35–45, and over 65) for each national group is presented in Table 8-2. The Japanese, Korean, Thai, and Taiwan samples inferred the greatest physical pain for the youngest age group, with next highest ratings for the oldest age group. The Puerto Rican sample also inferred the greatest pain for the youngest age group, but the next highest rating was for patients in the middle age group. The sample from the United States inferred the greatest pain for the oldest age group, followed by the next highest ratings for the youngest age group.

The United States, Japanese, Puerto Rican, and Taiwan samples inferred the greatest psychological distress for the oldest age group and the middle age group. The Korean and Thai samples inferred the greatest psychological distress for the middle age group, followed by the oldest age group.

Interaction Between Sex of Patient and National Group

The fourth hypothesis predicted an interaction between sex of the patient and national group. The analysis of variance for ratings of physical pain and two sex variables for each different culture resulted in significant differences among national groups for males (at $p \leq .001$) females (at $p \leq .001$) and significant differences between males and females for ratings of physical pain (at $p \leq .01$). For ratings of psychological distress, the differences for males and females were significant (at $p \leq .001$), but the difference between males and females was not statistically significant. Thus, the fourth

Table 8–2
Mean Ratings of Three Age Groups for Each Country

| Country | Age Groups | | |
	4–12	35–45	65+
United States			
physical pain	3.02	2.96	3.03
psychological distress	4.18	4.47	4.65
Japan			
physical pain	3.82	3.63	3.74
psychological distress	4.36	4.78	4.78
Puerto Rico			
physical pain	3.18	3.03	2.97
psychological distress	4.54	4.90	4.97
Korea			
physical pain	3.96	3.73	3.75
psychological distress	4.56	5.03	4.94
Thailand			
physical pain	3.31	3.11	3.18
psychological distress	4.03	4.62	4.54
Taiwan			
physical pain	3.63	3.40	3.59
psychological distress	3.63	4.23	4.34

hypothesis, which predicted an interaction between sex and culture, was supported for physical pain, but not for psychological distress.

A summary of the means of physical pain and psychological distress ratings for the two sex variables for each different national group follows in Table 8-3. Mean ratings of physical pain for both male and female patients showed the same pattern for all national groups. Female patients were seen as suffering greater physical pain. The Korean sample inferred the greatest difference between males and females, followed by the Japanese, Taiwan, Thai, Puerto Rican, and United States samples. Mean ratings for psychological distress in both male and female also showed the same pattern for all groups. The greatest difference was for the Korean sample, followed by Puerto Rican, Japanese, United States, Thai, and Taiwan samples.

Summary of Results

The results of this research strongly supported the general hypothesis that nurses from various countries differ in their inferences of suffering. This was true for inferences of both physical pain and psychological distress. In addition, significant interaction effects were found between national group

Table 8-3
Mean Ratings of Two Sex Variables for Each Country

Country	Male	Female
United States		
physical pain	2.95	3.06
psychological distress	4.39	4.47
Japan		
physical pain	3.70	3.76
psychological distress	4.57	4.70
Puerto Rico		
physical pain	3.02	3.10
psychological distress	4.75	4.86
Korea		
physical pain	3.79	3.82
psychological distress	4.76	4.92
Thailand		
physical pain	3.14	3.26
psychological distress	4.36	4.43
Taiwan		
physical pain	3.46	3.62
psychological distress	3.99	4.14

and each of the following variables: nature of illness, severity of illness, and age of patient. A significant interaction between national group and sex of patient was also found for ratings of physical pain, but not for psychological distress.

Discussion

This study began with the assumption that attitudes about suffering were, in part, socially learned responses. The results incontrovertibly confirmed this assumption. Nurses from one culture were markedly different from nurses from another culture in their inferences of physical pain and psychological distress. Each of the cultures studied revealed a distinct pattern of beliefs about patient suffering.

Empathic Quality

Among all cultures studied, Korean and Japanese nurses consistently inferred the greatest patient suffering for both physical pain and psychological distress. This finding was extremely interesting in view of the fact that, from the point of view of many people in Western societies, Orientals are thought of as stoic and presumably less sensitive to pain and distress. For example, in a study of American nurses' inferences about the suffering of patients with various ethnic and national backgrounds, Oriental patients were consistently seen by Americans as experiencing less pain and less emotional distress than any other groups. Davitz and Davitz (1974), in their *Extensive Progress Report* of the suffering study, state: "In general, for both dimensions of suffering, nurses see Jewish and Spanish patients as suffering most, and Oriental and Anglo-Saxon/Germanic patients as suffering least" (p. 82). This was interesting in comparison to the result of this study. At least two groups of Oriental nurses, the Korean and the Japanese, believed that patients in their own countries suffer significantly more than American nurses believe American patients suffer. These results provided dramatic evidence of the importance of one's point of view in making inferences about another person's experience. Obviously, the point of view of American nurses differed a good deal from that of Japanese and Korean nurses, and this difference was reflected in their inferences of patients' pain and psychological distress.

These findings raised an interesting question about relationships of American nurses and their Oriental patients. If American nurses believed that Oriental patients suffered much less than other patients did, it was possible that American nurses might have been inattentive or somewhat less sensitive to the distress experienced by their Oriental patients. However, if the results obtained from the Korean and Japanese nurses in this study reflected a cultural characteristic that can be generalized to Orientals in the United States, perhaps these patients were in fact more, rather than less sensitive to pain and psychological distress. If this is the case, American nurses might have been relating to Oriental patients from a point of view that was, in some respects, the antithesis of the patients' own perspective. As a result, the nursing care of these patients may have been less than optimal. Obviously, the results of the present research did not provide direct evidence about this issue. These data were, of course, obtained in the respective countries of the various groups of nurses, and there might have been important cultural differences between, for example, a Japanese patient in Japan and a Japanese-American patient in the United States. Nevertheless, the results of this study strongly suggested further research along this line, investigating possible differences between the experiences of Oriental patients and the inferences American nurses would make about these experiences.

The differences between the common Western stereotype of the stoic Oriental and the result obtained for the Korean and Japanese nurses might reflect determined beliefs about the relationships between behavior and experience. In the American culture, it may be assumed that behavior and experience relatively agreed with each other. If a person was indeed suffering, an American nurse might have very well expected that person's behavior to express his or her suffering. Similarly, if a patient was not overtly expressing distress, the American nurse might have assumed that he or she was not likely to have been experiencing distress. In other words, American nurses, reflecting their own cultural background, might have assumed a parallel relationship between overt behavior and experience.

This relationship between behavior and experience was certainly different among certain Oriental cultures, such as the Japanese and Korean. Among the Japanese, for example, control of overt emotional expression was valued, and from a very young age, children were taught to inhibit overt expression of their feelings of distress. At the same time, intensity of emotional experiences and sensitivity of feelings at an experiential level was also highly valued in Japanese culture. Thus, in contrast to the American's expectation of congruence between behavior and emotional experience, the Japanese might have assumed a certain degree of incongruence, particularly with respect to the expression and experience of suffering. This difference in assumptions about the relationship of overt behavior and experience may have been a source of difficulty in communication between members of these different cultures.

Although Korean and Japanese nurses ranked at the top of all groups in inferences of suffering, Taiwan nurses consistently ranked in the middle for physical pain and were the lowest in terms of psychological distress. Although Oriental, the beliefs of Taiwan nurses clearly differed from those of Japanese and Korean nurses. This finding underscored the fact that all Oriental cultures can not be meaningfully clustered together for all purposes. From a Western perspective, there may have been some tendency to view all Oriental groups as essentially the same, regardless of the particular countries involved. With regards to inferences of suffering, at least, the result of this study demonstrated that Oriental national groups differ among themselves just as one would expect groups from various Western countries to differ.

Among the cultures studied, the Puerto Rican sample showed the lowest inferences of physical pain and the second highest in terms of psychological distress. This finding was in accord with a previous study by Davitz and Pendleton (1969a). Once again, the results of the Puerto Rican sample reflected a unique cultural pattern or style. On the basis of the present study, this style cannot be fully explicated; however, the data suggested an interesting pattern that might be followed up in further research. Although there are wide individual differences, in the Puerto Rican culture people were generally expected to be emotionally expressive. For example, in contrast to a Japanese patient, a Puerto Rican patient might be expected to express his or her feelings more openly and perhaps somewhat more dramatically. However, the results of this study suggested that, while Puerto Rican nurses might have tended to discount these overt behaviors as expressions of physical pain, they also tended to believe that their patients were in fact experiencing a high level of psychological distress. Thus, the assumed relationship between overt behavior and experience for Puerto Rican nurses was different from that of the American sample as well as the Japanese and Korean samples. For the Puerto Rican sample, overt behavior may be assumed to parallel psychological distress, but not necessarily physical pain. Thus, in a culture in which patients were presumably expected to be relatively more expressive (in contrast, for example, to Japan), the behavior may be assumed to reflect primarily psychological distress rather than physical pain. Further research will be needed, of course, to clarify this proposition.

The sample from the United States showed the second lowest ratings for both physical pain and psychological distress. The relatively low degree of suffering inferred by these nurses might be attributed to the fact that the majority of the American sample were from Anglo-Saxon/Germanic backgrounds. According to Zborowski (1969), the perceptions and expressions of Old American patients were somewhat different from Jewish or Italian Americans. He states:

> The clinical impressions of medical practitioners that patients of Jewish and Italian origin tend to be more emotional while experiencing and expressing pain than the Anglo-Saxon—that is, the Old American—was confirmed by the observations derived from our study. Emotional description of pain experience occurred more frequently in the interviews with the Jewish and Italian patients than with the Old American and Irish. This emotionality was also expressed in the tendency of the Italian and Jewish patients to emphasize their perception of pain (to play up pain), whereas the Old Americans and Irish tended to deemphasize their perception (to play down pain).

The nurses from Anglo-Saxon/Germanic backgrounds in this study might have reflected the same characteristics as the Anglo-Saxon/Germanic patients in Zborowski's research. Thus, the low ratings for physical pain and psychological distress by the American nurses in this study might have represented a cultural tendency "to play down pain." In future research, American nurses from other cultural backgrounds should be studied to determine whether or not the tendency to infer relatively little suffering is particularly true for Anglo-Saxon/Germanic nurses or is a more general American phenomenon.

Body and Mind

In the ratings of the differences between physical pain and psychological distress, the Taiwan sample showed the smallest difference, followed by the Korean and Japanese. This may have reflected a general Oriental belief about the relationship between body and mind or between physical and psychological concepts. From this point of view, physical and psychological phenomena were intimately related, even though experience and behavior may not closely parallel each other. In contrast, the samples from the United States and Puerto Rico showed the largest differences between ratings of physical pain and psychological distress. At this point, it is difficult to interpret this finding with a great deal of confidence; however, further research might profitably explore this difference as a function of cultural beliefs about the relationship between physical and psychological phenomena.

Beliefs about Illnesses

Korean nurses showed the highest ratings of both pain and psychological distress associated with trauma and psychiatric illnesses. This may have reflected their experiences with patients injured during the Korean civil war. As a result of the war, these nurses may have worked with a relatively large number of patients suffering from traumatic injuries or psychiatric disorders, and as a consequence, they may have been especially sensitized to the suffering associated with these kinds of conditions. Japanese nurses inferred the greatest suffering for cancer in terms of both physical and psychological dimensions. According to a public health report published by the Ministry of Health and Welfare of the Japanese government in 1972, cancer was the second leading cause of death in Japan. Once again, this may have reflected their relatively greater experience with patients who have cancer, and their special sensitivity to the suffering associated with this illness. On the basis of the present study, one can only conclude that nurses in the several national groups sampled viewed the suffering associated with particular illnesses and conditions somewhat differently. Perhaps this reflected some difference in their professional experience with these illnesses; future research might consider these possible differences.

Sex Differences

It was particularly interesting to note that regardless of culture, women, in comparison to men, were seen as suffering more physical pain. This might, in part, be a function of the fact that all of the participants in this study were women; female nurses might be particularly sensitive to the pain of female patients. However, the results might have also reflected a more general belief that women were more sensitive to pain than men.

Although the samples in this study identified women as suffering more physical pain than men, there were no differences among cultures on the psychological dimension. Thus, although women were seen as more sensitive than men to physical pain, the nurses in this study did not believe that women differed from men in terms of psychological distress.

Age of Patients

Nurses from Oriental countries, Japan, Korea, Thailand, and Taiwan, saw patients in the oldest age groups as suffering more than patients in any of the other age groups. This might be related to the fact that in Oriental societies, respect and care for the elderly is a fundamental responsibility of all members of a given society. Thus, nurses in an Oriental culture might be especially sensitized to the suffering of elderly patients. Nurses in the United States also saw elderly patients as experiencing a relatively high degree of suffering. This finding may be a reflection of increasing concern for the elderly person in the United States and recent emphasis of programs to deal with the health care needs of patients in this age group.

Addenda

In addition to the six countries reported in this study, further data was collected from professional nurses in Uganda, Nigeria, Nepal, England, Israel, Belgium, and India. The English version of the questionnaire was distributed to nurses in Uganda, Nigeria, and India. Nurses in these countries are required to be fluent in English. The only substantive changes made were the omission of first and surnames for the hypothetical cases. Patients were simply designated as male and female. The reason for this change was to eliminate possible bias. In India, Nigeria, and Uganda, names may indicate tribal, caste, or social class affiliation. Preparation of the questionnaire for the other languages, for example, Hebrew, French, Nepalese, followed the three step process. Bilingual nurses translated the *Standard Measure of Inferences of Suffering* questionnaire from English into the other language. Another bilingual nurse back-translated the questionnaire into English. The two versions were compared for accuracy. The final questionnaire was duplicated in the United States and sent to the other countries for distribution. Nursing leaders in each country served as liaisons, arranging for volunteer subjects, distribution of the questionnaires, and the return of the completed questionnaires to the United States. The examples in Figure 8-1 show how one question appeared in six of the different languages.

Analysis of the data from all thirteen countries confirmed the assumption that attitudes are, in part, socially learned responses. Nurses from one culture markedly differed from nurses in another culture in their overall inferences of physical pain and psychological distress.

Among the thirteen cultures, Korean nurses inferred the greatest psychological distress, Puerto Rican nurses were the second highest, Ugandan third. Nepalese, Taiwan, and Belgian nurses inferred the least amount of psychological distress (see Table 8-4).

Among the cultures, Korean nurses inferred the greatest amount of physical pain for patients described in the questionnaire. Japanese nurses were second, Indian nurses third. Nurses from Belgium, the United States, and England inferred the least amount of physical pain (see Table 8-4).

An important implication of this study is the appreciation and recognition of markedly different cultural responses to inferences of physical pain

Figure 8-1 Question #7 in Different Languages

ENGLISH

	None	Little	Mild	Moderate	Great	Severe	Very Severe

7. After a series of tests and examinations, Catherine Kent, forty-two years of age, was hospitalized with thrombophlebitis. Therapeutic measures include anticoagulants and bedrest.

	None	Little	Mild	Mod-erate	Great	Severe	Very Severe
Physical Pain, Discomfort:	1	2	3	4	5	6	7
Psychological Distress:	1	2	3	4	5	6	7

HEBREW

שאלה 7

כאב גופני ואי-נוחות: 1 2 3 4 5 6 7

מצוקה נפשית: 1 2 3 4 5 6 7

7. לאחר סידרה של בדיקות ואיבחונים, אושפזה קתרין קנט, בת ארבעים-ושתיים, עקב דלקת-ורידים פקקת. האמצעים הטיפוליים כוללים תרופות נוגדות-קרישה ומנוחה במיטה.

JAPANESE

7. 一通りの検査の結果、42才のアクロマリン
さんは静脈血管血栓症と診断され
入院させられた。治療は安静と抗
凝固剤の投薬である。

肉体的苦痛	1	2	3	4	5	6	7
精神的苦しみ	1	2	3	4	5	6	7

Figure 8-1 (continued)

CHINESE

7. 康太太五十九歲，在經過各項試驗及X—光檢查（後診斷）其患忠血栓性靜脈炎，故住院接受及抗（凝血劑）藥物治療及臥床休心。

身體方面之疼痛，不舒服：　1　2　3　4　5　6　7

心理方面の之不適：　1　2　3　4　5　6　7

NEPALESE

शारीरिक पीडा तथा असुविधा　१　२　३　४　५　६　७

मानसिक पीडा　१　२　३　४　५　६　७

FRENCH

7. A la suite d'une série de tests et d'examens, Catherine Isseri, âgée de quarante deux ans, a été hospitalisée pour thrombophlébite. Les mesures thérapeutiques comprennent anticoag-ulant et repos au lit.

Douleur Physique ou Malaise　1　2　3　4　5　6　7

Angoisse Psychologique　1　2　3　4　5　6　7

Table 8–4
Mean Ratings for Each Country

Country	Mean Psychological Distress	Mean Physical Pain
Korea	4.84*	3.8062*
Puerto Rico	4.80	3.06
Japan	4.63	3.72
Uganda	4.60	3.60
India	4.54	3.68
Nigeria	4.53	3.39
United States	4.43	3.00
Thailand	4.39	3.20
England	4.36	2.81
Israel	4.29	3.25
Belgium	4.16	3.00
Taiwan (Formosa)	4.06	3.53
Nepal	3.60	3.56

*The higher the rating, the greater the psychological distress or physical pain inferred.

and psychological distress. It is interesting to note that Korean and Japanese nurses inferred both great physical pain and psychological distress particularly in view of the fact that many people in Western societies think of these Oriental groups as stoic and less sensitive to suffering. In our study concerned with ethnic background of patients, American nurses, for example, rated Japanese and Korean patients as having little pain or distress. However, when Japanese and Korean nurses rated Japanese and Korean patients, the perception of suffering was quite different.

According to a Japanese colleague, Westerners cannot 'read' Japanese people. She stated that "as little children, we are taught not to show feelings on our faces. We will smile for the world, but inside we may feel great despair."

The differences among Korean, Japanese, Thai, Chinese, and Nepalese nurses were striking. When we presented these findings to a group of nurses, one commented "Weren't you really comparing Oriental and Western societies?" For her, and for some Westerners, Oriental people are part of one group. The results of this study demonstrated that Oriental national groups differ among themselves just as one would expect groups from various Western societies to differ. In America these differences aren't always recognized and there is a tendency to stereotype the stoic Oriental as if all Orientals were alike.

Among the cultures studied, the Nepalese nurses and Chinese nurses were the lowest with respect to judgments of psychological distress. We talked with Nepalese nurses and Chinese nurses in the United States about this finding. According to them there is much less emphasis placed in their culture on interpretations of feelings. One Nepalese nurse noted, for example, that in Nepal the study of psychology of behavior and motivations for nurses was certainly not prominent in the curriculum. A Chinese nurse added that she believed that Chinese people did not have the inner 'turmoil' she felt many of her American friends seemed to experience. The explanation offered by the Chinese nurse was quite different from the interpretation of the Japanese nurse who stated that whereas children are taught to inhibit overt expressions of distress, at the same time intensity of emotional experiences and sensitivity of feelings on an experiential level were highly valued in Japanese families.

The Puerto Rican nurses rated psychological distress of patients very high and physical pain very low. Obviously, our data cannot explain this finding, but we might share the interpretations of the findings that several Puerto Rican nurses offered.

"We know our people are very emotional. We are always expressing what we feel—singing, dancing, laughing—so if someone is in the hospital we know they feel very upset but they might not have much pain. When I take care of a Puerto Rican patient, I expect them to tell me how terrible they feel. They do feel bad, no matter what is wrong with them. Just because they complain a lot I know they might not really be in pain. I am used to Puerto Rican people being very dramatic about themselves."

It is particularly interesting to look at the ratings of Jewish nurses for Jewish patients in Israel. Relatively low degrees of suffering for both physical pain and psychological distress were inferred. In our study of American nurses' beliefs about the suffering of patients from different ethnic backgrounds, the American nurses judged Jewish patients' suffering among the highest of any ethnic group. In interviews with American nurses from non-Jewish backgrounds the reactions were that Jewish patients were more demanding and expressed their suffering more than any other group of people. However, this contrasts sharply with the opinions of Israeli nurses dealing with Israeli patients.

The samples from Belgium, the United States, and England had the lowest ratings for physical pain and about the same for psychological distress. English nurses, among all the cultures, were the lowest for physical pain. According to some researchers, individuals from Anglo-Saxon/Germanic backgrounds tend to play down pain. In our talks with English nurses at the time of the study working in the United States, we were repeatedly told that one of their major adjustments to patients had been the fact that people in America had such little tolerance for pain. They talked about English patients having resiliency and strength. As one told us, "British people do keep a stiff upper lip." Certainly, in terms of our findings, British nurses inferred little pain in patients and little more psychological distress.

The findings from this study provide dramatic evidence of the importance of one's point of view in making inferences about another person's experiences. The results also raise important questions about relationships of nurses to patients. If nurses from one culture hold a particular set of beliefs about another culture, do these beliefs influence the nature of care? To what degree does stereotyping of another culture influence professional practice?

Important implications result from this study for American nurses, who perhaps more than nurses in the other cultures studied, will come into regular contact with people from a variety of ethnic backgrounds. Our interviews with nurses revealed innumerable instances where they found themselves reacting strongly to what they felt were unwarranted reactions to situations. For example, if a nurse was from an Anglo-Saxon/Germanic background and tended to minimize physical pain and psychological distress as our findings indicated, how did her beliefs influence her treatment of individuals from Korean or Japanese backgrounds? The external behavior of these people might not have indicated the depth of their feelings and thus meaningful relationships between nurse and patient were blocked simply because of vast differences in cultural orientations.

We certainly do not propose that nurses discard their belief systems and become 'universalists' in their thinking. We do suggest, however, that understanding our belief systems about suffering, the cultural patterns which are part of our thinking, can provide us with insights that will help us to deal effectively with patients whose values and attitudes differ from our own. An important consequence of the recognition of cultural differences with respect to beliefs about suffering can prevent a great deal of misunderstanding, misperceptions and lead to more effective, sensitive patient care.

9

A Comparison of Inferences of Suffering
Made by Black and White Nurses

In a previous study concerning the effect of ethnic and racial background of the patient on nurses' inferences of suffering, some attention was paid to the nurse's own background. However, the sample of nurses obtained in the earlier study did not provide an adequate basis for evaluating the possible effect of the nurse's background. The present study was undertaken, therefore, to determine whether or not the nurse's racial background makes a difference in inferences of suffering. Specifically, the purpose of this study was to compare the inferences made by black and white nurses with reference to both black and white patients. The major question of this research was: Did black and white nurses differ in their inferences of physical pain and/or psychological distress? In addition, the research considered a possible interaction between race of the nurse and race of the patient. That is, did black nurses differentially evaluate the suffering of black and white patients? Did white nurses differentially evaluate the suffering of black and white patients? If these differences exist, was the pattern of ratings different for black and white nurses?

Method

Subjects

The subjects of this research were 152 nurses at the time of the study working in one of three large metropolitan hospitals. Of the total sample, 76 were black and 76 were white. Within the black sample, 38 nurses rated black patients and the other 38 nurses rated white patients. Similarly, within the white sample, 38 nurses rated black patients and the other 38 rated white patients.

The four subgroups in the sample were: white nurses/white patients;

white nurses/black patients; black nurses/white patients; and black nurses/black patients. In each sub-group the majority of nurses were either staff nurses or head nurses, and their principal area of nursing was medical-surgical. The nurses ranged in experience from recent graduates to those with more than 20 years of nursing experience. In each sub-group, however, the majority of nurses had between one and 10 years of experience. In terms of position, area of nursing, and years of experience, the four sub-groups were very similar to each other.

Procedure

Each nurse who volunteered for the study was seen during the regular working day at the hospital in which he or she worked. The general nature of the research was described and the nurse was asked to fill out the *Standard Measure of Inferences of Suffering* described in a previous section. Instructions for this instrument were modified slightly for this particular study. Within the sample of black nurses, a randomly selected half were informed that the patients described in the instrument were black. The other half of the black sample were informed that the patients were white. This information was contained on the instrument received by each nurse, indicating that the patients he or she was asked to evaluate were either black or white, depending upon the particular subgroup to which that nurse had been randomly assigned. The same procedure was followed for nurses in the white sample.

Results

The average ratings for each sub-group for both physical pain and psychological distress are presented in Table 9-1. As indicated in Table 9-1, there was very little difference in the ratings of physical pain made by nurses in the four sub-groups. The analysis of variance showed that black and white nurses did not differ significantly in their inferences of physical pain and there appeared to be no consistent difference as a function of the race of the patient.

Table 9–1
Average Ratings of Physical Pain and Psychological Distress
for Comparison of Black and White Nurses

	White Nurses/ White Patients	White Nurses/ Black Patients	Black Nurses/ White Patients	Black Nurses/ Black Patients
Physical pain	2.87	2.99	3.07	3.01
Psychological distress	4.42	4.44	4.72	4.77

The results for psychological distress were somewhat different. In general, black nurses inferred a greater degree of psychological distress in patients than did white nurses, and this difference was statistically significant at the .05 level. However, the race of the patient did not appear to influence the nurses differentially. That is, black nurses, in comparison to white nurses, inferred greater psychological distress regardless of whether the patient was black or white. The crucial variable in this case, therefore, appeared to be the race of the nurse rather than the race of the patient.

Discussion

These results are of interest both in terms of the significant difference found for ratings of psychological distress and the non-significant findings for the interaction of nurse's and patient's race. On the basis of the present data, we cannot interpret with confidence the fact that black nurses tend to infer greater psychological distress than do white nurses. Perhaps this reflects broader sub-cultural differences between the two groups sampled. For example, within the black subculture in the United States, perhaps illness and injury is associated with greater psychological distress than it is within the white subculture. There is no direct evidence to substantiate this possibility, but it does suggest an avenue to follow in future research. The difference obtained between the black and white samples considered in this study may indeed reflect differences between nurses in the two racial groups, or it may reflect differences between the two racial groups that go beyond nursing. Without further investigation of this particular issue, the question obviously cannot be resolved. Nevertheless, the finding of a significant difference between black and white nurses with respect to inferred psychological distress opens up a potentially important line for further research.

The absence of a consistent interaction effect between race of the nurse and race of the patient was particularly noteworthy in view of the recent history of racial tension within the broader culture in which these nurses work and live. The results indicated that neither white nurses nor black nurses responded differently, at least insofar as inferences of suffering were concerned, to white and black patients. For physical pain, the degree of physical pain inferred appeared to be essentially the same regardless of either the race of the nurse or the race of the patient. For psychological distress, black nurses inferred a greater amount of suffering than did white nurses, but this was true for both black and white patients.

In this research we have dealt with only one limited aspect of nursing: inferences of suffering. Therefore, we cannot reasonably offer any conclusion regarding nursing practice in general. These results, however, were at least congruent with the hypothesis that white and black nurses did not respond differentially to white and black patients. Regardless of the tensions that may operate within the larger society, perhaps racial differences do not interfere significantly with the interactions between nurses and their patients. At this point, this proposition can only be considered a tentative hypothesis suggested by the results of this research, and it would certainly seem to be a hypothesis well worth testing in further investigations.

10
The Empathic Nurse

In the course of our research we had a chance to observe a large number of nurses who clearly provided very efficient and effective care for their patients. Among these excellent nurses, however, a relatively small group seemed to stand out from the rest. These were the nurses who were especially sensitive to their patients' feelings, took extra care and time in their relationships with patients, and seemed to provide an "extra" dimension of nursing care. In the more technical aspects of nursing their behavior was not very different from other excellent nurses we observed. They were efficient, obviously knowledgeable, and highly skilled. But their nursing was composed of something more than efficiency, knowledge, and technical skills.

From time to time we took the opportunity to talk with these nurses, and occasionally, to accompany them for awhile as they worked. Gradually, we came to recognize that the special quality characteristic of these nurses was a highly refined empathic response to their patients. They seemed to be very much "in touch" with their patients' experiences, particularly with regard to their patients' experiences of pain and psychological distress. We called this group "The Empathic Nurses."

Obviously, almost all of the nurses we have studied in our research have the capacity to empathize with the experiences of their patients. Thus, the Empathic Nurse did not have some unique quality that was not shared with other nurses. But it seemed to be a matter of degree; those we came to call the Empathic Nurses displayed a level of sensitivity that was, at least statistically, most unusual.

As a result of these informal observations we decided to study the unusually empathic nurse somewhat more systematically. The present study represents only a small first step in this direction. It was highly exploratory and was aimed only at discovering some possible further research. The results, therefore, must not be viewed as a basis for firm conclusions, but rather, as suggestions that may lead to further study. We studied this small sample of empathic nurses with the aim of generating hypotheses which could then be subjected to testing with further inquiry.

Selecting the Empathic Nurses

From the total group of medical-surgical, pediatric, and obstetric nurses observed in the three studies dealing with inferences of suffering and nursing behaviors (Chapter 8), ten nurses were selected on the basis of the following criteria: (1) high scores on the *Standard Measure of Inferences of Suffering*, and (2) high scores on the categories of observed behaviors that indicated active concern with the patient's feelings. These included, for example, exploring patient's feelings, expressing sympathetic understanding, and various nurturing actions. Thus, the ten empathic nurses we studied were selected on the basis of both test results indicating sensitivity to patients' suffering and observations of actual nursing behaviors reflecting active concern with patients' feelings.

The sample ranged in age from 22–55 years. Four were working on medical-surgical floors, three were in pediatrics, and three were in obstetrics. The group came from strikingly different ethnic backgrounds, for example, black American, Russian-Polish, Jewish, Italian, Irish, Puerto Rican, West Indian, Maltese, German, and Caribbean.

The Interview

Each of the ten empathic nurses was interviewed individually. These interviews were relatively informal and open-ended. The participants were told that we were interested in learning something about their backgrounds and their views of nursing, and after the initial question about why they entered nursing, the interviewer merely reflected what the nurse said or followed up any leads in the nurse's comments by open-ended questions, such as, "Tell me more about that," or "Could you explain that more fully."

The Findings

The results of these interviews were summarized in terms of the major themes that emerged from the nurses' comments. In each case, the theme was mentioned independently by at least seven of the ten nurses, and in some instances was discussed by all ten nurses. Thus, the findings reported here represent more or less common themes mentioned by the ten nurses who were interviewed.

Decision to Become a Nurse

In considering their motivation to enter nursing, there was no single motive or pattern of motivation that characterized this group. The reasons underlying their decisions to become nurses included a variety of factors, such as a search for a more meaningful life, a sense of responsibility to others, family encouragement, and chance.

My mother had to take care of the family by herself. My father died when I was nine. Even though we had very little ourselves, my mother always put aside some food for someone who might be hungry. She was always helping friends and relatives. I guess it was kind of natural that when I was ready to choose a career I would decide on one that let me play this role.

I come from a deeply religious family. They all had a tremendous responsibility to help others. Family duties and helping people were part of my upbringing. Several aunts were nurses and it was always understood in the family that I would follow them to England and train. The idea that nursing meant working with sick people, dealing with death and dying, never bothered me. I come from a culture where death is not feared. My mother had her clothes all ready for her burial even though she wasn't ill. Us kids knew about death. Death was part of our life. We even had prayers praying for death in our church.

My parents wanted me to go to nursing school so I'd have a profession. They helped me financially. When I graduated it meant a lot to them as well as to me. When I got my degree I had a great sense of accomplishment and the family—everyone—came to a huge party.

I was brought up in a rural area. My great-grandmother was a nurse-midwife. As a kid I often went with her to watch. I saw how much she meant to the women and how big a role she played in the lives of people. I might not have been aware of it at the time, but all this influenced my decision to become a nurse. I wanted to have the same kind of importance and respect. I knew I could achieve this with a career in nursing.

We were very poor. My family came to the States from Puerto Rico. My father got ill; my mother stayed home to take care of the kids. We were on welfare. Neither of my parents had much education. My father quit school in the fifth grade; my mother only went to the second grade. It was her dream that her children would have an education. My twin sister and I played nurse when we were small. My mother bought us nurse's kits. When we were fourteen we became volunteers at a hospital and were always called back because we were so reliable. Going to nursing school for both me and my sister was a natural step with all our experience as teenagers.

I went into nursing more by chance than anything else. I was the youngest of a large family. None of the others had gone on to school. I was the only one who expressed a desire. My parents had a real struggle getting together the $100 tuition. It meant a big sacrifice at the time. I really didn't know what nursing was all about. I wanted to go on to school and my two best friends had enrolled in nursing school. I just followed them.

I started as a psych. major in college. It was dull for me. It wasn't satisfying. I was drifting that year. About the middle of the term I happened to go to a career conference and talked with this dynamic, elderly woman. She struck me as very real. She was warm, wholesome, and I mean that in a positive way. I was impressed with her scholarship. She made sense and I went back to the dorm to think about what she had said. A couple of weeks later I went back to see her and told her that I had decided to switch to nursing.

I've always loved kids and I started out in school wanting to be a primary school teacher. I used to babysit a lot and I worked as a camp counselor. After I started practice teaching in a kindergarten I realized it wasn't for me. I didn't seem to be doing anything meaningful. I was really trying to find myself. I remembered a nurse who worked for a pediatrician I had gone to as a child and I thought about it for awhile and realized that if I wanted to work with children in a meaningful way that I should become a nurse.

I remembered when I was a kid I was sick and I had a nurse who was horrible. I know it sounds funny but the memory of her stuck with me and I made up my mind to go to nursing school and become the kind of nurse who cared.

I was a loner as a kid. I was interested in people but stayed by myself. I wanted to become an undertaker. I was quite serious about this. I thought that I could help people when they needed it most—families who had a death. I guess I thought more about death than most kids. When I was 12 my brother who was 8 was killed by a hit and run driver. My dad took it badly. Anyhow, I gave up the undertaker idea. I was married, had a child, divorced. For about ten years I supported myself and my child working on the stock exchange. I made good money, and I had a terrific career ahead of me. One day out of the blue I asked myself what is life all about? I felt I had to do something more meaningful with my life than work with columns of figures. I went back to school at night. And then the idea of becoming a nurse to help people crossed my mind. I made my decision and went into training.

Commitment to Nursing

Although the nurses in this group entered the field for a variety of reasons, once they became nurses, they were strongly committed to nursing. For them nursing was much more than the usual job; it was a central source of satisfaction, pride, and meaningfulness in their lives.

When I go to work, I feel good. I like what I do. I count in other people's lives and I never forget that for one minute. I feel very committed to nursing. Sure there are irritations but every job has problems.

Around the hospital they call me Little Florence Nightingale. I don't mind being teased. There's a lot of truth in what they call me. I have never lost sight of the fact that this is my life, my career. I'm not going to compromise myself or get embarrassed about being dedicated.

When I can't get into work, I feel guilty. Nursing isn't something you can do one day and then take off the rest of the week. People count on me. I don't feel I have the right to let them down. I try to get into work no matter what.

I love my work. I know that sounds corny but when I'm at work I feel like I'm in a 'bubble.' Nothing in the outside world comes between me and my job—my daughter, my husband, my family.

There never has been a single day when I haven't wanted to go to work. It's as simple as that.

Nursing isn't a 9–5 job. Sometimes it's more. I don't feel that it is a job because I get a sense of fulfillment about my days. Some of the girls think about just getting through seven or eight hours and then they can do something they enjoy. I don't feel like that. I enjoy what I'm doing.

The one person who did not share this sense of commitment had been a professional nurse for less than a year. Her feelings about work were mixed. On the one hand she enjoyed what she was doing, but the pleasure was tempered by the day to day frustrations she encountered. "It might be where I'm working, I'm not sure. Lots of things bother me like having to spend so much time with paper work—far more than the time I can spend with patients."

Nursing Education

Almost without exception, the group described their years in training as rigorous, demanding, and highly structured. Occasionally, they resented the demands and the discipline, but in retrospect, they talked about their experiences in nursing school with a great sense of pride. Having succeeded under the stressful and demanding conditions of their various nursing schools, they felt they could handle just about any challenge in their nursing career. Thus, their educational experiences were a significant source of professional confidence.

My school was very demanding. I can't remember one instructor who didn't know what she was doing. They were the most professional people I've ever met. The school never "slacked off." There wasn't a moment we weren't "hit" with the philosophy that if something was worth doing, it was worth doing well.

There was no leeway given to the student who was careless or sloppy. If a girl remained that way, she was dismissed. We had to conform to standards. I remember being constantly evaluated. There wasn't an aspect where we weren't judged—our manners, dress, behavior. There were no exceptions. I recall the demanding aspects of training; at the time I got angry. Some girls couldn't take it and left. Now I'm glad I stuck it out. I learned confidence. I think the nurses who aren't satisfied are the least competent.

I went to a school run by the Dominican Fathers. The sisters were Sisters of Charity. They had very high demands. Our skirts had to be two inches below the knees or we were reprimanded. They actually measured if there was a question. We weren't allowed to wear jewelry, makeup. The external controls imposed on the students helped us to gain internal discipline. We weren't allowed to let off steam. We had to have external controls no matter what we felt inside. I know that the way I act toward patients is because of my training. The school's philosophy was that patients must be treated with respect at all times. We were told over and over again that patients were individuals and must be reacted to with consideration. Patient needs were first and foremost.

My school was concerned with every part of our lives. Where I'm working, students will come on the floor having had only a cup of coffee and a cigarette at breakfast. I couldn't imagine anything like this happening to me as a student. Our matron (an English school) always gave us lectures about how we must start the day off with a proper breakfast. This is just an example of how everything that went on with students was a concern of the faculty. I'm sure that I gained considerable strength and discipline for having come up through a system that had very high standards of deportment and training.

My school was impossibly strict when compared to schools nowadays. I loved every minute of it. Maybe it was easier for me to accept than it was for some of the other girls. I had been brought up in a strict home where you had to obey your elders or else! The teachers at school actually were easier than my own family in some ways. We were checked constantly. We had to know our patients; we had to know what was going on; we couldn't get away with laziness, not caring, not knowing. If we didn't know something, it was up to us to find out.

My biggest memory of nursing school was being a lowly probie and holding my breath when the director of the school walked by. We were watched, kept in check. For the first six months we couldn't make a move without someone breathing over our shoulder. After the first six months we were given responsibilities. There was a dramatic shift and we were aware of the responsibility being given to us and the independence. I'm grateful for that kind of rigorous training I had. I learned confidence.

Only one woman reported attending a boring, mechanical baccalaureate program. She had found only one faculty member empathic to students' needs. "If it hadn't been for this one woman I probably would have left training. She was warm, sensitive, and loving. I can't ever remember her cutting a student down or cutting the amount of time she spent with us. But school wasn't very exciting. It was something to get through with as quickly as possible."

Role Models

Role models encountered during training or early in practice exercised an enormous influence on the majority of these nurses. In describing these models the nurses mentioned characteristics such as self-discipline, calmness, confidence, poise, and commitment. But regardless of the various characteristics mentioned, for most of these nurses there was someone in their backgrounds whom they viewed as an ideal nurse and whom they tried to emulate.

I vividly remember two people who made a big impression on me. I wanted to be like them though at the time it seemed impossible. Still in all, it didn't keep me from trying. One was the school director. It's been over thirty years since I was a student and I can still picture her, slim, blonde, always dignified and poised. She was so confident and assured. Sort of an immaculate kind of person if you know what I mean. She had a great way with the students. They all loved her.

Mac was a small, bustling Scotch woman. I don't know what we would have done without Mac. She backed us up. Her philosophy was that we could do anything if we tried. All of us wanted to very much to please Mac, not to let her down. Other staff members yelled, criticized us publicly—never Mac. She never raised her voice and if she had anything to say to us she made sure she talked privately. Mac was devoted to nursing and had such a 'jolly' attitude. I've never met anyone in all my experience who could make patients and staff feel so reassured.

I worked with Shirley my first year out of school. I used to watch her and hope that I would become like her. She could go from bed to bed, never losing her calmness, never getting uptight but doing things constantly to make patients happy.

The greatest impression made on me was by a supervisor. I used to marvel at the way she could take a staff member who had a problem and needed to talk and turn what could be an awful situation into a positive one. Her strength was unbelievable. She kept everyone going—helpful to the patients and everyone on the staff.

I always think about one nurse when things get tough and I've had it for the day. She was calm, dignified. I thought how great it was the way she could be such a ramrod of strength. She was dedicated. I wanted very much to win her approval and tried to be like her. I think I still do. I know I never lived up to her expectations at the time, and I'm not the sort of person who never breaks, but I keep trying. She made me feel so good about myself. Never did she let on that I had failed or did something wrong. She was the same way with everyone.

Although the vast majority of the group had been influenced through positive encounters with outstanding nurses, one woman stressed the impact "bad nurses" had on her performance. For this individual, observations of what she termed "poor nursing" made the greatest impression.

What I mean is that when I worked with a nurse who was hostile and mean to patients, I'd say to myself, "I'm never going to be like that no matter what." I've worked with staff who resented every minute on the floor. That bothered me. Again, I'd think to myself, "If that day comes, I'm going to leave nursing." It's not a matter of age, I've found out. I've met older nurses who are warm, kind, take the time to help younger nurses, who are great with patients. I've watched young nurses behave the same way. The hard angry ones can be old or young. It doesn't matter. I'm convinced it's the individual and not the age or anything else that makes a difference.

Self-Esteem

Perhaps the most striking and consistent characteristic shared by all of these nurses was their professional self-esteem. They knew they were good nurses and conveyed their self-evaluation, not with any sense of bragging or boasting, but with quite, secure confidence.

Nursing to me is a total kind of thing, not something I do only for money. Sure, I like to get paid for what I do, but I'm a nurse in uniform or out of uniform. What I am trying to say is that basically I respect that kind of person I am. I don't put on a uniform like a mask and turn on caring or whatever. I am myself at work or out of work and this makes a huge difference in how I feel about my job and myself. I know a lot of people can't wait until the end of the day and they can "become themselves." I am myself at work—the same kind of person when I'm out with friends or at home.

I happen to believe in myself and what I do. I know I have one fault which drives some people wild. I am a perfectionist. It doesn't bother me though because I'm not going to compromise my professional standards or my own standards for anyone or anything.

I feel sure of myself and what I do. Perhaps this is because I've come up the hard way. Maybe I would be different if I had had a middle-class background. I don't know. I've pulled myself up from the bottom and I know what it's like to come from a family on welfare and parents who had no education. I've been on the other side and I've accomplished a great deal. I respect what I've done. I don't mean I have to go around convincing people I'm somebody. I'm confident. This doesn't mean I still don't have a lot to learn.

I know where I'm going and what I'm doing. I never feel hopeless or helpless. There are plenty of times I don't know what to do or have doubts but I'm never at a total loss.

Respect from Colleagues

In addition to their self-esteem, these nurses were also secure in their sense of being respected by others. Thus, each nurse's self-concept as an effective nurse was reinforced by the evaluations of others with whom she worked.

In all the years I've worked I've never felt that doctors didn't respect what I do. Maybe it's the group I work with. I am free to make decisions. The doctors on the staff thank me. Many times they'll tell me to use my judgment, we trust you. When I have to telephone a doctor and tell him to come he responds immediately. He knows I wouldn't call unless it was absolutely necessary. I'm talking about the staff doctors. I know what I'm saying doesn't hold up always with some of the others who use our hospital facilities.

I'm not the kind of person who sits back and takes what is handed out from other people without a word. If I'm right, I'll stand up for my rights. No one can stand in my way. Doctors and other nurses know the way I am and they respect men. I treat them with respect and I've never failed to be treated in the same way.

I'm a fighter. If I'm right, I'll hold to my opinion. That bothers some people. But I do listen. If I'm proven wrong, I'm the first one to admit my error. I think because of the way I am, my co-workers and the doctors respect me. No one respects a person who lets herself be walked over. I'll have doctors ask my opinion. It's very important for me to have my judgments respected.

I know a lot of nurses complain about doctors not respecting them. I think I do have the respect of my co-workers. The fault isn't so much with the doctors I think as it is with the system. In my hospital we never have group discussions about patients. There are no chances to get together to discuss patients. The hospital respects the doctors but forgets about nurses' needs. I think that if we had a chance to sit down together as a group to review cases, there would be a huge difference in the kind of respect doctors had for nurses and the other way around.

Respect from doctors depends on the doctor. But then that's true with the other nurses. I think I'm respected even though I disagree a lot with other people. I feel pretty confident and sometimes people resent this, though they have to respect me for holding to my opinions when I'm right and they know I'm right.

My supervisor disturbs me the way she behaves towards the doctors. She shakes when they come around. I don't think they respect her more because she fawns all over them. I don't want to behave like that. I am not defensive. I know my job; I respect my colleagues and I want to be treated the same way. I think because I am sure of myself and I am not apologetic or submissive, I'm respected more.

Caring for Others

Caring for others was unquestionably the most important source of professional satisfaction reported by these nurses. They emphasized both the intrinsic reward they experienced in helping another person as well as the appreciation expressed by others.

My satisfactions in nursing come from working with people who are sick and seeing them get better and ready to go home. I like the feeling of being appreciated by the patients, that I helped make this possible. When they show they trust me and respect me, I feel good about myself and my work.

The most rewarding part of nursing is patient contact. I enjoy being looked up to by the patients. I enjoy relating to them in a personal sort of way. My greatest satisfactions come when patients welcome me. They feel I understand them. I like being thought of as someone special. I know this is a fact because I get feedback. There is laughter, conversation. Then many times others on the staff will tell me that so and so was asking for the nurse with the long braid. I get a glow of satisfaction when I hear this.

I get a sense of fulfillment about my days. The rewards for me come when I help someone. I know when patients express appreciation, a small gift, a box of candy, and there's nothing wrong with these things, I have a sense of achievement, well being.

I think there is nothing greater than a feeling of having helped someone. I think being empathic as a nurse is so important. There is a line between you and the patient but reaching out and knowing you have succeeded is a good feeling.

I enjoy being liked and needed. The satisfaction I get comes from my patients and this is very important for me. When I see a patient ready for discharge, standing up straight, getting ready to leave the hospital, and feeling good, I share the feeling.

Relating to Patients

Throughout the interviews, the nurse's relationship with his or her patient was repeatedly emphasized as the core of nursing. This central concept was expressed in a variety of ways, but in one way or another each of the nurses underscored the crucial importance of how he or she related to patients.

Some of the nurses talked about the time they devoted to their relationship with patients.

It gripes me to hear nurses talk about not having enough time to do the kind of job they want to. It's just an excuse. There's always enough time. Somehow you can find the time if you really care.

My biggest problem with patients is getting overwhelmed. My supervisor is always after me for being slow. I find I want to spend time with patients. I do what is necessary for each one and then go on to the next step. My supervisor doesn't see it this way. She is always hurrying everyone. Even though I get my work done, she says I'm slow. I really don't want to change. Caring for patients is what nursing is all about.

I think it's nonsense that nurses don't have enough time to be kind or caring. Even on the busiest days you can be sympathetic. When I'm rushed and can't take time I go back later in the day. No one would stop any nurse from going back to a patient when the nurse had more time. I think our profession would do itself a great service if we stopped blaming the clock for our behavior. It doesn't help the nurses or the patients to use time as a reason for the way we might behave.

A number of the nurses talked about the ways in which they related to especially difficult patients.

When patients are hostile I tell myself, they're not rational. It makes me angry when nurses reject patients they say are hostile or demanding. I have never yet failed to believe that a call is an honest call for help. It might not seem like that sometimes because of the kind of request or question the patient has. But there's a reason. It could be they're upset and need a little attention. I think I'm like a lot of nurses and I have problems handling psychological distress. It's a lot easier to handle the physical complaints. And I know that a call for psychological help is as real as anything else. One of my friends who is a nurse lost a baby. Everyone stayed away saying they didn't know what to say to her. I went in and we talked. She got a chance to tell someone how awful she felt. All she needed was someone to listen to her.

I never really become upset with hostile or demanding patients. It always flashes through my mind that the patient isn't accountable for what she might be saying or doing. In another situation that patient could be completely a different person. I think I can cope with patient aggression because I never take it personally. Some nurses do and that's a mistake.

Hospital patients never throw me. I know they are displacing their anger at themselves on to me. I always tell myself when I walk into a new patient's room and they are angry with me how could it really be me when they don't even know me. I know the patient is angry at being in the hospital. I never show anger in return.

Many of the nurses in this group emphasized their sense of respect and caring for patients.

> I respect my patients. I respect them and I want to be respected. I think my respect for patients comes from my training. I was taught that we always had time to put ourselves in the other person's place. I find many times thinking this could be my sister, my father, my mother. How would I want them treated?

> I have a child and I believe that if I behave in a caring way toward my patients, toward everybody, my child will receive rewards. This is part of my culture to think like this. I think that people from the Islands are more humanistic. American nurses seem much less sympathetic. They're caught up in the technical part of nursing and seem to forget people are in those beds and not machines.

> I respect every patient where I work. I know what it feels like to sit on a bench in an out patient clinic. I sat there many times with my mother or father. I know how awful we felt when some nurse was rude to my mother and I knew she was sick. I'll never behave that way. I know what it is like to be on the other side.

> In nursing school and at work we're always being told to distance ourselves from our patients. I don't agree. I don't think I could be a good nurse and not care. It's impossible to disassociate yourself from patients. I think of the way I behave as controlled disassociation. I have to care and yet I have to have control of my empathy or I can't do a good job.

> No matter what a patient says or does I keep trying and caring. It never fails to win a patient over. When I go into someone who is very sick and that person is rude or unpleasant, I look at the patient and ask myself how I would feel if that were me in that bed. How would I behave? Some patients are stoic and cheerful. Most people though give in more to themselves. When the situation is bad enough. When I think about how I would behave if it were me, I can't possibly do anything that would be hurtful.

Teaching

Although caring for others was the primary source of professional satisfaction, a second area mentioned by several nurses was teaching. Thus, they viewed as an important part of caring for others the process of teaching others to care for themselves.

> Teaching is a part of nursing that is very important to me. I enjoy teaching. It's not just enough for a nurse to go into a patient and do the necessary things. It's just as important to teach the patient to care for themselves.

I think patient teaching is the most important part of my work. I know that I enjoy this role very much. I could do with a lot less paper work. We write instead of teach. I think many nurses hold back, don't spend enough time instructing their patients. I know that I feel an obligation to my patients to explain procedures, to talk with them about what I am doing instead of engaging in a lot of idle chit-chat. Patients appreciate being taught.

Personal Lives

Life outside of nursing was described as very satisfying. They experienced normal ups and downs, but in general they expressed a sense of enjoyment in their friends, families, and activities outside of the hospital.

Nursing takes a big chunk of time in my life. I never resent it. I think a lot has to do with my family and friends. I'll meet someone and they find out I'm a nurse and they're impressed. My family thinks what I'm doing is the greatest. I guess I'm lucky this way. Lots of my friends have jobs they hate; they feel they aren't doing anything meaningful. One of my old high school friends keeps telling me she wished she had gone to nursing school instead of straight college. She ended up as a super secretary and can't wait to get out of the office.

My husband is very proud of me. He's always telling people he's married to a nurse. There's never been a time when he hasn't pitched in with the housework or taken care of the kids because I've been too tired. The extra income is important, but that's not all there is to it. I know he respects my being a professional.

I think part of why I enjoy what I'm doing is because it's not my whole life. I mean if all I had was nursing I don't think I'd be happy. It gets kind of depressing at times. But I have a good social life. I'm in no rush to get married; I have a steady boyfriend. We probably will end up getting married next year. But now both of us like the freedom.

It makes a big difference if you have other people in your life besides nurses and people from the hospital. I know that I count a lot on my family and friends. I think I'd be different if after work I went back to an empty house.

Discussion

In many respects, the nurses we talked to in this study were very different from one another. They came from widely different backgrounds, entered nursing for a variety of reasons, worked in a diversity of hospital settings, and their styles of personal life varied greatly. There were several interrelated themes that characterized their comments about nursing. These themes might be viewed in terms of commitment, confidence, and caring.

Commitment

Having entered nursing for many different reasons, once they became nurses there was no question about their dedication and commitment to nursing. In our conversations with them they were certainly not unrealistically idealistic or at all concerned with trying to impress us with their altruistic motivations. If anything we would characterize them as down-to-earth, practical-minded professionals. But it was clear, nevertheless, that nursing for them was much more than a mere job. It was difficult to capture the essence of all their comments; each of them was too much of an individual to fit into a single mold. Perhaps the closest we came was that, from their different perspectives, they viewed nursing as a "calling" rather than as just another job. In saying that they viewed nursing as a "calling," we did not mean to suggest any religious implications; however, for this group, nursing was a profoundly meaningful part of their lives. It was not the only source of meaning; by and large, their interests and activities outside of nursing were both varied and satisfying. But the values derived from nursing were extraordinarily important to them.

On the basis of our interviews, we cannot determine how this sense of personal and professional commitment developed. From their reports it did not seem that this commitment was present for most of them when they entered nursing. Rather, it developed during their training and later experiences as nurses. There does not appear to be a specific method of achieving this commitment. Each nurse in a unique way discovered the meaningfulness of nursing, and as a result of this gradual process of discovery, became increasingly committed to nursing as a central aspect of his or her life.

Confidence

In addition to a sense of commitment, each of these nurses clearly expressed confidence as an effective nurse. Thus, they not only enjoyed what they were doing, but they also knew that they were doing it well. This self-esteem was reinforced both by appreciation from their patients and respect from their colleagues.

Frankly, their comments about the demanding and structured nature of their nursing education at first surprised us. We had not anticipated this finding, though it became less and less surprising as each successive nurse in the course of our interviews independently described the rigor of training. We do not believe that the rigor of training in and of itself made these nurses especially empathic. Their training, however, contributed to their self-esteem and confidence, which permitted them to deal with the stresses of patient care without feeling threatened. They expressed a good deal of pride in the fact that they had successfully passed a very difficult course of training and felt that in this training they had acquired the personal and professional skills necessary to function effectively, regardless of the particular problems they encountered in their nursing careers.

Caring

There was never any question about the purely technical competence of the nurses we talked to; in fact part of their confidence was based on their secure knowledge of the more technical aspects of nursing care. But in discussing their views of nursing care, they went far beyond technical competence. They emphasized their own needs to care for others and the importance of their relationships with patients. They took the time to care, were not unduly disturbed by very difficult patients, and respected the people with whom they worked.

Of the many factors that contributed to the development of this general attitude toward patient care, the nurses in this group focused particularly on the influence of role models early in their nursing careers. Each of them had an opportunity to observe another nurse, usually a more senior person, who represented for them an ideal nurse, and the theme of caring was an important part of this ideal.

The Empathic Nurse

There is no simple way of describing or explaining the personal and professional development of an especially empathic nurse. It is much too complex a problem to be dealt with adequately in one very limited investigation. Nevertheless, the three interrelated themes of commitment, confidence, and caring would seem worth considering in further study. In this preliminary research, we feel that we have only scratched the surface of a very important problem, and the questions raised by this pilot investigation are far more significant than any tentative conclusions we might suggest. For example, how can nursing education foster and enhance a student's sense of commitment to nursing? Following the lead of the nurses we talked to, is a very demanding, highly structured, and rigorous course of training consistently related to the development of a sense of commitment and confidence? How can the conditions of nursing practice be designed to reinforce nurses' self-esteem and confidence? What are the factors in current practice that work against the development of professional self-esteem? How can nursing schools achieve an appropriate balance between emphasizing high level technical competence and recognizing the importance of interpersonal processes in nursing? Can we identify potentially important role models, and how can the impact of these role models be enhanced?

These are only a few of the questions raised by this preliminary study, and it is quite obvious that our research has resulted in many more questions raised than in answers even tentatively given. Addressing these questions in further research, however, may provide a systematic foundation for future advances in the education of nurses and the practice of nursing.

Part Four

Changes in Nurses' Beliefs

This section reports two investigations. The first is based on a series of interviews with a large number of graduate nurses who discussed their reactions to patient's suffering. The second study reported in this section deals with changes in beliefs about suffering over the course of nursing education.

11

A Natural History of
Nurses' Reactions
to the Suffering of Patients [1,2]

Up to this point the major thrust of our research had involved investigating a series of theoretically derived propositions concerning nurses' inferences of suffering. To supplement the experimental and correlational studies, the present research was undertaken with the aim of exploring nurses' reactions to the suffering of patients at various stages in a nurse's career. In contrast to our previous work, no specific proposition or hypothesis was tested. Rather, the purpose of this research was to describe the "natural history" of nurses' reactions at various points in their professional careers. It was hoped that, on the basis of this descriptive investigation, further variables relevant to the main line of our work could be defined and meaningful questions formulated for future research.

Method

Subjects

The subjects of this research were 203 nurses at the time of the study working in one of four large metropolitan hospitals. These nurses came from all major units in the several hospitals (e.g., emergency, obstetrics, surgery, pediatrics, coronary care, etc.), and their experience ranged from recent graduates to those with more than 20 years of experience. No effort was made

[1]A version of this study was reported in *The American Journal of Nursing*, September, 1975, pp. 1505–1520, entitled "How do nurses feel when patients suffer?" Copyright © 1975, The American Journal of Nursing Company. Reproduced, with permission, from *American Journal of Nursing*, September, Vol. 75, No. 9.

[2]The investigators wish to express their appreciation to the several Directors of Nursing, other hospital administrators, as well as the nurses who participated in this study. Without their cooperation, of course, this work would not have been possible.

to predetermine selection of subjects; the aim was merely to study as large a group of nurses as could be obtained within a reasonable period of time. Although systematic data were not available, our observations during the course of data collection suggested that the nurses cooperating in this study were a fairly representative sample of nurses working in large urban settings. There was no apparent systematic bias in the selection of subjects; however, it should be noted that all subjects were volunteers who were willing to devote at least an hour to a discussion of their experiences and feelings about the suffering of patients.

Procedure

Data were collected by means of small group interviews. These groups ranged in size from three to seven nurses, with a model group composed of five participants. The interviews took place in the hospitals in which the nurses were working and were held during the regular working day.

In every group meeting three general questions were posed for discussion. Participants were asked to think of a particular patient for whom they had felt a great deal of sympathy and to describe their reactions to the suffering of that patient. They were also asked to think of a patient for whom they felt less sympathy and to describe their actions and thoughts regarding that patient. Finally, they were asked to think about themselves during training as compared to the present. In what ways had they changed in their response to patients who were suffering? In what respects had they remained the same? The group interviews lasted about an hour, and the participants were encouraged to exchange ideas and to compare their views and experiences. Other than presenting the three general questions for discussion, the investigators did not guide or direct the interviews. Their comments during the course of the interviews were limited to reflections of feelings, brief questions asking for further clarification, and occasional summary statements.

Results

The content of these interviews has been categorized into the specific points raised in the various sessions. The order of presentation follows: first, a discussion of the differences between training and practice, the changes nurses noticed in themselves as they acquired greater professional experience. This leads to a discussion of the kinds of patients for whom they feel more or less sympathy, and their reactions to these patients. This is followed by a discussion of the complaining patient and the psychiatric patient, and difficulties in dealing with these patients. We then turn to the problem of a nurse's over-involvement with particular patients and the need of the nurse to maintain a certain amount of emotional distance. Finally, we present the nurses' comments about reactions to death and dying, a topic that evoked very strong and emotionally meaningful reactions among the nurses who participated in these sessions.

It should be kept in mind that this report does not test any theory or hypothesis about attitudes or behaviors toward suffering. We are not trying to *prove* anything. Our intent is to share ideas, problems, and issues raised by nurses. Thus, in presenting the various points, we are not suggesting that any single statement is necessarily true of all nurses in all places at all times. Rather, we are merely suggesting that the nurses' comments that are presented are well worth thinking about, and we hope that these excerpts will raise further questions and stimulate further research relevant to nursing education and practice.

From Training to Practice

Many of the nurses spoke about the differences between nursing school and actual practice, and the changes they have noticed in themselves as a result of their nursing experience. This change was often described as a shift from the idealism of school to the realism of practice, a shift from a kind of universal sympathy to more controlled and selective reactions.

I know I don't feel the same toward patients now than when I was a student. As a student I think I cared more because it was my whole life. Now I think I care differently because nursing is only part of my life. I don't cry or feel all torn up inside because a patient is suffering. In a way I'm a better nurse. As a student sometimes I felt my emotions kept me from behaving therapeutically.

As a student every patient was a crisis. Every patient was in great pain and suffering. It was my duty to help in the best way I could. That sure has changed. Now if a patient refuses my help or wants to leave the hospital, I don't beg them to stay. My attitude is, "You don't want us, then you can go."

In school I felt bad for everybody. (When I was a student) a chest pain and a sore throat were all disasters. If someone said their throat was sore, I rushed around. Lie down, rest, gargle, I couldn't do enough for a complainer with a sore throat. Over time I realize you have to react individually according to your own judgment.

I know a lot of teachers in nursing schools teach that it is OK to cry with a patient if that's the way you feel. There's nothing wrong with showing emotion. But I feel since I've been in practice restraint is important. You won't do the patient or the family any good if you stand there dissolved in your own tears.

Although most nurses talked about becoming more practical, realistic, and down-to-earth as a result of their professional experience, others reported an increased sensitivity to and emotional understanding of the suffering of others.

Nursing education, at least for me, was a matter of studying, memorizing, and analyzing. I was so busy being a student I didn't have time to feel. You have time to feel when you're in practice. I think over time, I'm a far more sensitive and compassionate person than I was when when I was in training.

Practice has made me softer. I think I was more calloused as a student—probably because there was so much going on and you think in terms of labs and courses—not people.

When I was a student I just assumed people suffered. That was it. I mean if you're a patient you have to expect to be in pain or worried. Now that I've been working for a couple of years, this really bothers me.

Perhaps the two aspects of change with practice, becoming more realistic and also becoming more compassionate and understanding, were explained by the increasing selectivity of nurses' reactions. This apparently began with the realization that patients were people, and people were different from one another. Thus, many nurses described their current reactions to patients in terms of a more selective sympathetic response in contrast to the universal empathy of their nursing school experience.

You get to realize that you don't feel the same about everyone. It's a rude awakening. I thought all people were nice. In practice, I've discovered all people aren't nice. Some are and some aren't. It's the same way with the saviour complex. When I went into nursing my idea was to save everyone. I realized you can't—you simply can't. Some people are going to die, no matter what you do.

I can hear my instructor now, lecturing on how you can't get annoyed, you shouldn't ignore a patient. You have to feel empathy for everyone. Reality has taught me I can't react to everyone in the same way.

When I first saw myself behaving differently, I got all upset. It wasn't right. But then you can't just treat people the same. For example, my first emergency room experience. When I first worked in the unit, a patient would say, "I've been here three hours." Oh my goodness, three hours. I would rush around and demand the patient be seen. My goodness, what right has that person to wait three hours? Now I see priorities. You can't start worrying about a sore throat in an emergency room when police are bringing in victims from an auto accident. You start with people in that accident. The others can wait three hours or four, if necessary. Some people are suffering more than others.

Differences in Reactions to Patients

Each nurse was especially sympathetic to certain kinds of patients. Some responded particularly to the young, some to the old, others to those who reminded them of parents or friends.

I think we all have favorite patients—kinds of people who trigger off a special feeling. I know old people who don't complain get to me. And then young kids if they're not too way out in their behavior—lonely patients. These kinds make me feel something inside.

I have an idea that most nurses I know are more torn apart when you work with young patients who have serious illnesses. Young people are very disturbing. It isn't fair they should suffer. I feel for the parents. I guess I could compare my feelings for parents of children in for tonsillectomies. If they carry on, I turn off. But when I have a seriously ill child with concerned parents the situation can be traumatizing.

Different kinds of people do turn you on. I mean, the fact is some people just get a rise out of you and others are just there to be taken care of. I get a different feeling when someone my own age comes in or someone reminds me of my parents, or even friends.

The nature of the illness made a tremendous difference in the nurse's reaction. The nurse responded most strongly to those who were likely to die or be severely disabled; by and large, much less sympathy was felt for patients with minor illnesses and those who didn't have a "legitimate" basis for complaint.

I just can't feel the same for a patient who let's say has an appendicitis and one who has cancer. They are different and I know the person who is post-op for appendicitis might have pain; still, in all, I really feel bad for the person who has cancer. Maybe I say to myself that the patient with appendicitis is going to be OK. In a few days he'll be fine. It isn't true for cancer. It's only going to get worse. Knowing this makes me more sympathetic toward that person.

I just couldn't feel anything for this woman even though she had a great deal of pain. This was her sixth operation for beauty's sake. When she complained I couldn't see her pain as being real. She did it to herself for her appearance. I know I made her wait before I responded. How can you feel anything for someone who is so spoiled and vain that she will go through surgery six times?

Sometimes the nurse's own personal experiences made a significant difference in her response to particular patients. Having gone through experiences similar to those of a patient, a nurse may be especially sensitive or "tuned in" to a patient's suffering.

I've wondered if you feel more for a patient's suffering if you've gone through a similar experience. I think about myself. Before I had a baby I worked in labor and delivery. We'd have these women carrying on as if the world were coming to an end. 'Come on now,' I felt like telling them. 'You're putting on a show.' Well, let me tell you, I had a baby and I had a difficult labor. You ought to see me now on the floor. All that a woman has to do is squeak about her pain and I empathize right with her. I think you just have to have had some experiences or you can't really have any idea how a person feels.

For most nurses, a feeling of sympathy for the patient led to increased contact with that patient. They were more likely to stop in and just chat with that person. In contrast, there was much less conversation with patients for whom they felt little sympathy. By and large, except in the case of a dying patient with whom the nurse was strongly involved, the amount of conversation a nurse had with a patient was probably a good indicator of the degree of sympathy the nurse felt for that person.

With patients I feel something for I'll talk about anything. I can always find something to talk about. With someone I don't feel anything for I don't even talk about the weather. I simply say, "Do this or that"—I keep conversation at a minimum.

When I go in to a patient for whom I just can't feel much of a reaction, I don't say more than I have to. I feel guilty because the patient sometimes will try to talk and my responses are terse. I say just what is necessary—not a word more.

Nurses realized that it was not merely what you say to a patient that makes a difference, but how you say it. Thus, the communication between nurse and patient involved both verbal and nonverbal components.

I know from myself and listening to other nurses that something changes when you talk to patients you care about and to those you don't. When you sympathize with a patient, I think—I know I do—you speak more slowly. There's a tenderness in your voice. You don't run out of the room. If the patient wants to talk, you stay and talk. Or maybe you don't talk at all because you don't know what to say, but there's something in your face that lets the patient know you're pulling for him.

Something happens to you when you're with patients you feel a lot for. I think it's like a wave of gentleness or tenderness. It sweeps over you when you care. I suppose I show it in my voice and hands. I know that inside I feel warm and soft. I'm sure I do something to express that feeling.

There are ways of saying things. I will say to one patient, "Just ask for your pain medication once"; I sound really sarcastic. But this was a patient who never asked once but dozens of times and she just turned me off.

The Complaining Patient

Nurses had certain expectations regarding patients who had a "right" to complain, and those who were merely "complainers." There was a crucial difference between those patients whom the nurse believed were really suffering and those who were seen as overreacting and complaining simply for the sake of complaining.

> I feel I know who is sick and who is making a noise. Then I realize I treat people who I feel are really sick different from the way I do people who are just making a noise.

> I react negatively about people, people who overreact. It bothers me when I feel a patient can't really be in all that pain and they insist on reacting. I think it's unfair to spend time with people who carry on without a good reason when I should be spending my time helping people who are really in pain and much quieter.

Continuous repeated complaints, if they were seen as unwarranted, were frustrating, and for the nurse constantly faced with these complaints, irritation, annoyance, and anger were not uncommon responses.

> I am irritated with patients who complain about everything. I have found that most of these people aren't sick at all. The really sick ones who need you don't complain. When I get an idea that someone is just exaggerating, I am annoyed. I feel those patients take me away from someone who needs me but is quiet about it. I resent the others. They make me angry.

> When I don't feel sympathy for a patient simply because I know they are not really suffering, I still do what I have to in terms of care, but I think I sound angry. I know I stay at the foot of the bed of those people. I never go up to the head of the bed. I hear myself talking a mile a minute and then I walk out without waiting for an answer.

> Sometimes a patient will turn you off. They aren't all that sick and they complain and are always at you for this and that. I get angry inside. I don't yell or scream, but I realize my voice lowers in pitch. I may sound angry. It worries me the patient will know what I'm feeling. I try to catch myself when I feel this way.

In addition to feeling angry, the nurse typically avoided the over-complainer. Some nurses talked about delaying their responses to the complaining patient's call. Others responded, but didn't hear what the patient said. In a variety of ways, they tried to escape from the over-complainer.

> If I think a patient is putting on a light just for the usual complaint, I don't think I see it. I'm not conscious of the light. With complaining patients I know I wait longer to respond. I don't rush into the room.

> I can't really sympathize with the patient who is constantly putting on her light or calling for a nurse. Get me this, do that, they're never satisfied. After a while, when you get a patient like this, you want to stay away because you know

nothing seems to make them happy. They think they are in a hotel and talk about services or they just want you to stay at their bedside and wait on them.

There are some patients I don't hear. I know they're talking and asking questions but I can't hear a word they're saying.

Simply trying to fulfill the over-complaining patient's demands usually didn't help matters. The complaints just went on.

Every so often you get a patient who I am sure lies in bed making up demands. I've been called to pick up a tissue box that was right next to the patient. From my experience the demanding patient is never satisfied. It seems the more you fulfill the demands the more is demanded. It's a vicious cycle.

Nurses may or may not have expressed their anger openly, but when they recognized their own feelings, they frequently reported a sense of guilt about these feelings, regardless of whether or not they have expressed them.

I feel guilty because I know the patient is sick and maybe not responsible for his actions. I can't help not liking the patient but I also feel guilty. Then I go into the patient's room and try to make it up to them.

I may lecture to patients. I know when I go into a long harangue about something the patient should do, what is happening is I'm trying to make up for negative feelings.

Dealing with Emotional Problems

In some ways related to the problem of dealing with overly complaining patients was the issue of working with patients who had psychiatric or emotional problems. Particularly for some nurses not involved in psychiatric nursing, patients with emotional problems tended to elicit relatively little sympathy.

I guess I don't feel much sympathy for people with psychiatric problems. I mean they come in neurotic, all upset, and self-centered. I don't want to take care of them.

Of course, I take care of these people. I give them attention and I try to sympathize with their problems but deep down inside of me I wonder about why they can't get on top of their problems.

Part of the nurse's difficulty in dealing with emotional problems was feelings of helplessness or inadequacy in relieving this kind of suffering. The nurse could have administered medication to reduce physical pain, but didn't have similarly effective and efficient techniques for relieving psychological distress.

> It's so much easier to cope with physical pain than psychological suffering. If someone has physical pain you can do something and you see the results. I know that's why I prefer the recovery room to the med-surg floor. I feel satisfied when I can help. But on other units you had to handle physical pain *and* psychological problems. I had compassion. I feel for most of the patients, but honestly I haven't any idea what is best to do. If someone is depressed or is disturbed, what do you say? What can you do? You can't handle it the way you handle physical pain.

> We studied psychological theories and practice and counseling techniques but in practice you don't sit down with a patient an hour a week or everyday in one hour sessions. I learned all sorts of involved techniques. The fact is you haven't an hour to spend with a patient. Nowhere in school did they tell me how to be therapeutic in five minutes. We work on schedules. The morning hours are hectic. Perhaps on night duty you have more time, but then patients go to sleep or have their own evening visitors. I feel I'm beginning all over again and haven't any guidelines to help me cope with psychological problems.

> Something has happened to me in the years since I've been out of school. I know I've become more aware of psychological needs. As a student I never thought about the psychological needs except in psychology classes. But now I'm more aware and concerned. It bothers me that I can't do more to help patients who have psychological problems.

The Problem of Over-Involvement

Far more common than the problem of avoiding over-complainers was the other side of the coin—the nurse's sense of being overwhelmed by the very real suffering of patients he or she worked with everyday. Nurses described a variety of reactions to this stress, including, for example, the empathic development of physical symptoms that parallel those of a particular patient.

> I had this one patient I was caring for on the floor for several months. I really felt for this patient and there were times when I actually felt like I had the same symptoms. I really had chest pains. They were so bad I had myself checked out. Nothing was wrong and I realize now I was so upset about the patient that I started to get the same kind of pains she had.

> Lots of times when I have patients that really upset me because they're in such pain or maybe depressed or worried, I get physical reactions. I've had headaches. Then there was this woman with thrombophlebitis in her legs and she was suffering terribly. I remember feeling my legs hurt whenever I had to go into her room.

The effects of daily experience with the suffering of others was felt not only at work, but also when the nurse left the hospital. Nurses often reported they found themselves taking patients' problems "home with them."

> I'm drained when I get home. If I've spent a day feeling for other people, I get frustrated. My family gets the worst side of me. I can get explosive, angry, and when someone at home sounds off about they're sick or worried, I get resentful. I ask myself, who is going to listen to my aches and pains?

> I have lost contact with old friends. Now I'm more comfortable when I'm with people in medicine. They have more to say to me. You see I feel as a nurse I've touched the real cores of life. This makes you wake up. Other people can go along—and never see what I see. I grew up in practice far more than friends my own age who aren't nurses.

> If you like being a nurse it's twenty-four hours, whether you like it or not. I have called co-workers at night to talk about a patient who worried me.

For many nurses, sometime after they began practicing they realized the need to develop some emotional distance between themselves and their work, some defense against over-involvement.

> I think you have to block out some of the patients' suffering. If I reacted to every patient, felt deeply, I couldn't exist outside of the hospital or in the hospital for that matter of fact.

> I don't take sides. All patients are patients to me and I don't react. I just don't let myself get emotionally involved either way.

> I couldn't take the pain and suffering when I first started to work. My work history is horrible. One year on and one year off, or sometimes three months at a stretch. It's better now but simply because I've built up some defenses.

Frequently, the realization of a need for emotional distance developed as a result of experience with a patient for whom the nurse felt especially sympathetic, and who subsequently died—leaving the nurse feeling drained, traumatized, and ineffective.

> I was very tired. Taking care of him had been very exhausting emotionally and physically. I realized later I couldn't get attached this way for my own sake. The next couple of weeks I kept a certain distance between myself and other patients. If I didn't, I knew I couldn't give the kind of physical care they needed. Giving so much of yourself emotionally interferes with physical care.

> I've learned that it isn't a good idea to let yourself care too much about one patient. I feel that you aren't being effective when you let yourself get car-

ried away emotionally. I remember one time when a young woman died. The whole staff fell apart. We were all so broken up by her death that all the other patients on the floor weren't taken care of. It isn't fair to the other patients when one individual means so much.

Thus, to maintain their own emotional stability and remain effective in professional practice, nurses built psychological defenses against over-involvement. These defenses typically involved establishing some emotional distance between the nurse and patients. But specific defensive reactions took many forms, including, for example, seemingly macabre but psychologically meaningful hospital humor.

I think we (*nurses*) build up defenses about suffering. I think we depend on humor. Maybe it isn't humor—more like black comedy. I know there are some awful situations when people make jokes. To an outsider the humor would seem terrible, but in the hospital it's very funny. I guess humor helps you cope.

Reactions to Death and Dying

Of all the daily problems encountered by nurses, the death of a patient was emotionally most devastating. Even after years of professional experience, nurses described their reactions to the death of a patient with whom they had worked in terms of feelings of helplessness, depression, anger, and despair.

I was caught up with the patient. He was in terrible pain and very worried about his family. He didn't ask for anything—just lay there staring. I tried to get him to talk but he shook his head and yet I had the idea he wanted me to stay in the room. I felt awful. Inside, the pit of my stomach felt ripped. I was nauseated. He didn't have a chance to live. I think he knew it and I knew it and I got very depressed.

It's very hard right after a patient dies and you've really spent a lot of time and cared what happens. For days it seems like I have a dead weight on my back.

When I was a student it was a lark. I was going to help people. I was young and had never seen a person die, a baby being born. It was a game I was playing. Now it's real. In school we were protected even from death. I can recall how we (students) were rushed away one afternoon because a patient was dying. Now each day I see more and it's been depressing.

I remember his clothes were shabby and he had only a few dollars in his wallet. I could picture his life—he had come to the big city to make it and he was going to die. He hadn't even had a chance and there was no one who knew him or who cared. We went into the bathroom and cried. I had his wallet—just a card and a few dollars.

The notion of death depresses me. I can't solve the problem. I'm not afraid of dying patients. I try not to be, but it is always a haunting experience.

I keep asking myself, what did I do, what didn't I see? Couldn't anything have been done?

I had a 23-year-old patient who didn't want to die. We fought with her. We fought and she fought but we were helpless. She wanted desperately to live. She hung on to us every time we came into the room. What do you do? How can you be supportive? What can you say? I think about her. I didn't run away at first and then it was my first time with a dying patient. I wanted to get away. She died and couldn't be revived. I thought to myself, what good am I in a situation where I can't be effective? And then I felt anger. There's no damn need for a 23-year-old to die.

The death of young people was especially traumatic for many nurses.

I was taking care of a young girl who should never have died. She was demanding and kept calling me on the dictaphone. One afternoon she asked me to call her husband; she just wanted to know if he was OK. I got upset myself because when she was dying I started to cry—couldn't control myself. The supervisor got enraged. She said to me, 'You have no business crying. This isn't the first and last dying patient you will take care of.' I keep thinking even now—what right did she have to say that to me—to tell me how to feel? When she died I couldn't touch the body. I could look but not touch her. I was too shaken. The day nurses came in and washed the body and I stayed away from the room.

It makes me angry when a child dies. Why should a child die? Why should a young person die? I can't answer and it bothers me a lot.

It's hard. When you care the most it seems harder to know what to do. I had a patient recently, a young girl who was dying. Her mother was in the room with her—never left the child's side. The child was in a coma and the mother showed me pictures of how she looked when she had been well. I didn't know what to do to help her. There wasn't anything to be done to save the child. I dreaded being in that room.

When a patient with whom the nurse had been closely involved was dying, one of the most common reactions reported was a desire to escape from the situation—though physical escape itself often did not relieve the nurse's own sense of emotional distress.

She wanted desperately to live. She was in a tent and when you went near the bed, she would grab you by the wrist. She hadn't energy to eat by herself and her grip was unbelievable. She kept saying, "I don't want to die. I don't want to die." I couldn't bear going into the room.

> What can you tell someone? They ask if they are going to live. You know they aren't; the doctor knows—maybe the family knows. The only person in the dark is the patient. I can't answer. All I can think about is escaping.

> The last thing I wanted was to be on duty when he died.

The trauma of death was reduced somewhat when the patient was elderly and the nurse senses that the person was "ready to die."

> A 77-year-old man was very sweet to the end. He told us how he felt. "I'm ready to die," he said. "I wish they'd let me go in peace." He was much easier to nurse. I wasn't helpless. We prayed together. But as he said, "My job in the world is done." I just loved talking to him. All the nurses did. He was very calm. He asked us to shave him and help him get dressed. Imagine, and he died that afternoon. It was as if he knew that the hour was coming and he wanted to be clean and ready. I knew I had helped him—had stayed with him—done things, and I was glad that I had been able to be supportive.

In addition to nurses' immediate emotional reactions, the experience of the death of a patient also affected nurses' thoughts and feelings about their own deaths and reflections about themselves and their lives.

> I feel empty inside, part of me is gone and not coming back. Each time this happens I get a new awareness of myself as an individual who is also going to die. Then I say to myself, what I do in life from day to day is very important. If anything, encounters with death have increased my self-awareness.

> I think about life after I die. What's going to happen. I don't know. I'm not sure where I stand. Some people think there's a life after death—others don't. I've been entertaining the possibility of life after death more and more as I practice.

> The spectre of death is in the hospital. The time factor of life bothers me. As a student you plan for the future; you think in terms of saving, then in practice you wake up to the fact that you can't save some people. When I hear the call of 1-2-6, I shudder—I feel terrible. I realize I don't want to die.

> I think I've been able to learn to handle most situations, at least I hope so, but the one thing I haven't conquired is my reaction to death. I even think I can deal some with other people and their families but then I think about my own.

Discussion

The comments of the nurses and the implications of what they said raise many questions about nursing education and practice. We cannot hope to touch all of the issues raised, and we certainly don't intend even to suggest possible solutions. But we would like to underscore some of the central issues discussed by the nurses who participated in our groups, and perhaps suggest some questions that might be considered in dealing with these issues.

The Idealism of Training and the Realities of Practice

Many young people enter nursing with a strong sense of idealism that is reflected in a kind of universal sympathetic reaction to everyone who is suffering. This is certainly a very positive motivation for nursing, and in certain respects, it would be highly desirable to maintain this sense of idealism throughout a nurse's professional career.

But for some nurses, at least, the realities of practice provide a sharp jolt to this idealism. They cannot spend time with everyone who complains, they cannot relieve the suffering of every patient, they do not feel honestly sympathetic for everyone, and they cannot prevent death in every case. Thus, the initial idealism of their nursing school days is inevitably modified.

In and of itself, this process of modification is not necessarily undesirable. It might be viewed as part of the process of growing up as a professional nurse. Nevertheless, one cannot help but wonder about the degree to which nursing school experiences might foster an idealism that is incongruent with practice. With the recent emphasis on psychological understanding of the patient, has there also been an adequate parallel emphasis on understanding of the nurse? Do nursing students learn that patients are people, that some people are likeable and others are not, some people are cooperative and others are disruptive? Do they learn that nurses, too, are people—and that no person can like or feel sympathetic towards everyone? Is it always wrong for a nurse to feel angry? Should they feel guilty when they can't respond sympathetically? How do a nurse's feelings influence the effectiveness of nursing care? What can nursing schools do differently to bridge the gap between training and practice, idealism and reality, and the professional and human sides of being a nurse?

The Difference Between Reactions to Pain and Psychological Distress

Nurses see a clear distinction between the task of relieving pain and trying to comfort a patient suffering psychological distress. In the relief of pain, medications and other physical techniques are available. Though not always perfect, by and large they are relatively effective—certainly more consistently effective than the psychological techniques currently used to deal with emotional distress. Thus, nurses experience much more difficulty in responding to psychological aspects of suffering than to physical pain.

This difficulty is not because nurses are insensitive to or fail to understand the psychological dimension of suffering. Rather, it is primarily because effective and efficient techniques for reducing psychological distress are not readily available. As the nurses in this study pointed out, a general nurse working in a typical large hospital simply doesn't have the time or opportunity to spend long daily sessions with each patient, searching for profound, in-depth insights, and psychological understanding. This kind of continuing, long-term contact with patients is obviously unrealistic. Yet, it is precisely from a field involving such interactions, psychotherapy, that nursing theory and techniques for dealing with emotional distress have largely been derived. The differences between the psychotherapeutic and the typical nursing situation are enormous, and perhaps the theories and techniques developed for psychotherapy are inappropriate sources for the task facing a nurse. In most non-psychiatric situations, the nurse needs to deal with a patient meaningfully in a very brief time, not with the aim of effecting long-term therapeutic change, but for the purpose of relieving immediate emotional distress. What sources are more appropriate for the development of such techniques? Instead of searching for other sources, would it be more profitable for nurses and nursing researchers to focus on the problems and situations specific to nursing and develop techniques particularly suitable to the typical nurse-patient interaction? Should the structure of nursing practice be changed to deal with this problem, perhaps introducing specially trained nurses to work with the emotional difficulties patients experience? These are not new or novel questions, and we certainly have no answers, but they obviously involve issues of crucial importance in the improvement of nursing care.

Over-Involvement and Emotional Distance

The nurses in this study dramatically described the dangers of over-involvement with particular patients. In fact, it was often an experience of over-involvement with a specific patient that led the nurse to realize that deeply personal and emotional reactions can interfere with effective functioning.

Many nurses reported dealing with this problem by developing certain professional defenses, the most common of which is to maintain a degree of emotional distance from the patient. But this, too, involves dangers and difficulties. From the patient's point of view, the nurse may be seen as uncaring, rejecting, mechanical, adding to a patient's sense of loneliness and helplessness. From the nurse's point of view, work may lose some of the human quality that originally attracted the person to nursing. As a result, the nurse may become increasingly dissatisfied and even bored by the more routine and administrative tasks that permit the nurse to maintain a certain emotional distance from the patient.

Nurses have been concerned with this problem for a very long time, and there is no easy solution. Nevertheless, there are questions relevant to this issue that need to be explored, and perhaps in the process of exploration, a more adequate solution to this central conflict in nursing will be developed. For example, what is the relationship between emotional distance and nursing effectiveness? Is the nurse's sense of sympathetic involvement with a patient a condition of effective nursing care? In what ways does the structure of the hospital situation itself exacerbate this problem? How do the nurse's working relationships with other professionals influence the nurse's relationship with a patient? In what ways can the situation be altered to improve the interpersonal conditions of nursing for both the nurse and the patient?

Death and Dying

Recent efforts by nursing administrators and educators to deal more directly and openly with nurses' reactions to death and dying can only be reinforced by the results of this report. Of all the problems discussed by the nurses participating in this study, their reactions to the death and dying of patients clearly elicited the strongest emotional responses. We cannot meaningfully add to what the nurses have already said with such clear emotional force. Perhaps the only conclusion that needs to be drawn is a reaffirmation of the necessity to continue, and even expand, our concern for those who face the fact of mortality in their everyday professional lives.

12
Changes in Inferences of Suffering during the Course of Nursing Education

Previous studies in this line of investigation considered graduate nurses in a variety of settings. Thus, generalizations based on this research could be made only to graduate nurses who had some experience in professional practice. The present study was designed to expand this range of subjects to include nursing students. Specifically, this study investigated changes in inferences of suffering made by students during the course of their nursing education.

Interviews with graduate nurses suggested that nursing students' reactions to patients' suffering changed as the students gained clinical experience (see Chapter 11). These data were retrospective, however, and thus subject to possible distortions that might have occurred after the nurses who participated in these interviews had completed their education. Nevertheless, it seemed reasonable to expect some changes in beliefs about suffering as a consequence of nursing education.

By and large, students entering nursing education have not had a great deal of experience caring for people who have been ill. One could reasonably assume that they have had the normal range of experience with illness themselves and among members of their families as well as friends, but in most instances this probably involved only minimal contact with the degree of patient suffering that nurses routinely encountered in hospital practice. Thus, the beliefs about suffering held by entering students were probably based largely on cultural stereotypes shared by the population at large and had very little foundation in first-hand observations of people who were seriously ill.

When they enter nursing education, these students come into contact with people's physical pain and the psychological distress associated with illness. For some of these students this may be the first time they have had more than casual experience with hospitalized patients. Moreover, as these students progress in their education, they are given increasing responsibility for the care of patients and thus are faced with the professional task of dealing with the suffering experienced by patients with whom they work. Their beliefs about suffering, therefore, are no longer based primarily on cultural stereotypes, but are inevitably influenced by their own first-hand observations of patients as well as by the attitudes, beliefs, and behaviors of of nursing faculty, clinical supervisors, and graduate nurses working in training settings.

In addition to clinical experience, academic course work in almost all schools of nursing deals with various aspects of patient suffering. Both pain and psychological distress are considered in textbooks, lectures, and informal as well as formal class discussions. Thus, the nursing student not only has contact with patients who are experiencing pain and psychological distress, but is also exposed to more academically oriented considerations of suffering that accompany illness.

As a consequence of their clinical experiences, their academic studies, and contacts with faculty and nursing staff, students' beliefs about suffering were bound to undergo some change. At the outset of this research, however, the specific nature of this change could not be specified. There was no substantial theory to guide a reasonable prediction and little previous research that would provide a strong empirical basis for formulating specific hypotheses. Therefore, while some change in students' inferences of suffering was anticipated and predicted, this research was designed primarily as a descriptive study aimed at describing the pattern of changes that occur during the course of nursing education. Furthermore, assuming changes were found, a secondary aim of this research was to identify possible variables in nursing education that might account for the observed changes.

Method

The design of this research included both longitudinal and cross-sectional aspects. Longitudinal changes were evaluated over the course of one academic year by testing students early in the fall, soon after school for that academic year began, and then testing the same students again in late spring, shortly before the end of the academic year. Cross-sectional comparisons were based on testing students at each year level in the respective schools. In addition, data were also obtained for a sample of nurses who had graduated less than a year before the testing was conducted.

Subjects

Six schools of nursing participated in this study. Two of these schools offered associate degree programs, two offered diploma programs, and two offered baccalaureate degree programs. All six schools were in the New York-New Jersey metropolitan area.

School 1. One hundred ninety-eight students in school 1 participated. Of the 110 first-year students tested in the fall, 100 were retested in the spring. Of the 88 second-year students tested in the fall, 70 were retested in the spring. Because of absences and school schedules, not all students tested in the fall were available for testing in the spring.

School 1 offered a two-year associate degree program within a community college setting. The total program was composed of 65 credits; 31 credits were in nursing and 34 credits in basic sciences, psychology, sociology, etc.

School 2. One hundred fifteen students in school 2 participated. Of the 70 first-year students tested in the fall, 51 were retested in the spring; and of the 45 second-year students tested in the fall, 37 were retested in the spring. Once again, absences plus the school schedule prevented retesting all students who participated in the fall.

School 2 offered a baccalaureate program within a university setting. During the first two years in the program students enrolled for 64 credits in science and the humanities. No nursing courses were given during this period. During the final two years students enrolled for 46 credits in nursing. Thus, the first-year students tested in this research are juniors in the program, but in their first year of actual nursing education. And the second-year students were seniors in the program, but in the second year of nursing education.

School 3. One hundred twenty-six students in school 3 participated in this research. Of the 75 first-year students tested in the fall, 47 were available for testing in the spring. Of the 51 second-year students tested in the fall, 43 were available in the spring.

School 3 was a hospital school of nursing offering a two-year diploma program. The curriculum was composed of 28 credits in the sciences and humanities taken at an associated community college, plus 56 credits in nursing.

School 4. One hundred seventy-six students in school 4 participated. Of the 93 first-year students tested in the fall, 52 were available in the spring; of the 83 second-year students tested in the fall, 56 were available in the spring.

School 4 offered a two-year associate degree program within a community college. Students enrolled for 39 credits in the sciences and humanities and 32 credits in nursing. However, by far the greatest amount of time in the program was devoted to nursing.

School 5. Two hundred eleven students in school 5 participated. Of the 73 first-year students tested in the fall, 63 were retested in the spring; 70 second-year students were tested in the fall and 59 retested in the spring. All 66 third-year students tested in the fall were retested in the spring, with the addition of two students who had been absent for the fall testing.

School 5 was a hospital school of nursing offering a three-year diploma program. Students enrolled for 34 credits in the sciences and humanities and 58 credits in nursing.

School 6. One hundred eighty-three students in school 6 participated. Of the 40 first-year students tested in the fall, all 40 were retested in the spring, with five additional students who had been absent for the fall testing. Of the 82 second-year students tested in the fall, 66 were retested in the spring. Sixty-one third-year students were tested in the fall, with 28 available for the spring testing.

School 6 offered a baccalaureate program as part of a private, four-year liberal arts college. The nursing program was designed to cover a period of three years. During this time, a student enrolled for approximately 32 credits in psychology, sociology, etc., and the remainder of the program was devoted entirely to nursing.

Graduates. Fifty-eight nurses who had graduated less than one year prior to testing and who were currently working in one of four metropolitan area hospitals were also tested. This sample was composed of nurses who had graduated from each of the three types of schools represented in the sample of students.

Summary. A total of 1,014 nursing students in six schools of nursing participated in this research. Of these, 466 were in their first year of nursing education, 419 were in their second year, and 129 were in their third year.

Procedure

The *Standard Measure of Inferences of Suffering* was used to obtain the basic data of this research. Early in the fall of the academic year in which data were obtained, a team of researchers met with all students in each of the six schools. After obtaining informed consent of the students, data were obtained by group administration of the *Standard Measure of Inferences of Suffering*. The same procedure was followed for obtaining data from the sample of graduate nurses.

Interviews. In addition to the test data, 20 students from each year level in each of the six schools were interviewed with regards to their academic and clinical experiences relevant to patients' suffering. These were group interviews, with 4–6 students participating in each group. Each interview was approximately one hour in length.

These data were obtained for exploratory purposes to identify variables of potential interest for future research. Because of the exploratory nature of this aspect of the study, the interviews were relatively unstructured and open-ended. Students were asked to discuss how their nursing education had influenced their reactions to patients' suffering and to indicate how these reactions had changed during the course of their education. These interviews were conducted after the fall testing.

Curricula. Information about the curriculum of each school, including both academic and clinical aspects of the program, was obtained by examining the catalogues, bulletins, and other duplicated material provided by the administration of the participating schools.

Results

The basic data of this research were the average ratings of physical pain and psychological distress for each student over the 60 items in the *Standard Measure of Inferences of Suffering*. The first issue addressed in the analysis concerned differences in ratings over the course of education. Combining the data obtained cross-sectionally (in other words, at each year level) and that obtained longitudinally (in other words, at fall and spring testings), mean ratings were obtained for six points in the course of training (first-year fall, first-year spring, second-year fall, and so on) as well as for the sample of graduates. These results are presented graphically in Figure 12-1.

For ratings of physical pain, a one-way analysis of variance showed results that were significant beyond .001. The ratings of first-year fall students differed significantly from all other groups. Similarly, an analysis of variance of ratings for psychological distress obtained results which were significant beyond .001. Once again the ratings of first-year fall students differed from all other groups.

These results were obtained by combining data collected cross-sectionally as well as longitudinally. Exactly the same pattern of findings were obtained by separate analyses of the cross-sectional data (first year vs. second year vs. third year vs. graduates) and the longitudinal data (fall vs. spring for each year).

Inspection of Figure 12-1 reveals that, for both dimensions of suffering, changes in ratings occur during the first year of nursing education, but the changes for pain and psychological distress are in opposite directions. Inferences of physical pain decrease sharply between the fall and spring of the first year and then remain at about the same level throughout the period of education and during the first year of practice. In dramatic contrast, inferences of psychological distress increase sharply between the fall and spring of the first year, continue to rise during the second year, and then remain approximately the same throughout the period of education and during the first year of practice.

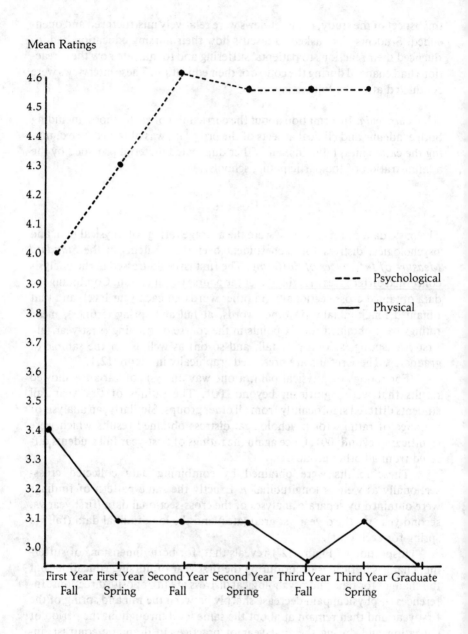

Figure 12–1
Mean Ratings of Patients' Suffering at Several Points in
the Course of Nursing Education

Thus, with regard to the central issue of this research, the data incontrovertibly demonstrate that inferences of suffering change significantly during the course of nursing education. Moreover, the results indicate that these changes occur primarily during the first year of training, and changes for the two aspects of suffering measured in this research are in opposite directions. Inferences of patients' physical pain decrease over the course of nursing education; inferences of psychological distress, on the other hand, increase.

Differences Among Schools

Pain. To evaluate differences among schools, a two-way analysis of variance, with schools and time as the independent variables, was computed. Mean ratings of pain for each school and for each stage of education are summarized in Table 12-1. The main effects for schools and for time were both significant beyond .001. The interaction between school and time was also significant beyond .001.

Inspection of Table 12-1 reveals that students in the six schools entered nursing education with different beliefs about patients' pain, and the pattern of change in these beliefs varied from school to school. For example, students in School 3, a hospital school of nursing offering a two-year diploma program, entered nursing school with, by far, the highest inferences of patient pain. By the spring of the second year, just prior to graduation, students in this school reported the lowest inferences of patient pain. Thus, there was a dramatic difference in pain ratings made by entering and graduating nurses in this school.

In contrast, ratings of students in School 5, a hospital school offering a three-year diploma program, were virtually the same at all stages of training. Students entered this school believing that patients in general did not suffer a relatively high level of pain, and students graduated from this school with essentially the same beliefs regarding the level of patient pain.

A detailed study of the demographic characteristics of the students and the curricula of the two schools did not reveal any variables that might account for the differences found for ratings of pain. Both schools were located in a suburban area, emphasized clinical experience throughout training, and attracted students from essentially the same general population. The first-year students in School 3 were somewhat older than those in School 5, which might have partially accounted for the higher ratings in the fall of the first year, but it seems unlikely that a small difference in average age would have accounted for a substantial amount of the variance in ratings of pain.

The patterns of ratings among the six schools were considered in relation to the degree offered (diploma, associate, baccalaureate); the setting (hospital, community college, four-year college or university); location (urban, suburban); and characteristics of the curriculum (for example, amount of clinical experience at various stages of training). None of these variables appeared to be consistently related to the pattern of beliefs about pain

Table 12-1
Mean Ratings by Students from Six Different Schools
at Various Stages of Education including Graduate Nurses

| | | First Year | | Second Year | | Third Year | | Graduate |
	Ratings	Fall	Spring	Fall	Spring	Fall	Spring	
School								
1 Associate	physical pain	3.02	3.08	3.25	3.11			
	psychological distress	4.22	4.35	4.76	4.71			
2 Baccalaureate	physical pain	3.32	3.27	3.18	3.27			
	psychological distress	4.18	4.13	4.56	4.47			
3 Diploma	physical pain	4.44	3.00	2.96	2.87			
	psychological distress	3.20	4.33	4.38	4.24			
4 Associate	physical pain	3.32	3.13	3.06	2.98			
	psychological distress	4.32	4.28	4.68	4.14			
5 Diploma	physical pain	3.15	3.09	2.97	3.13	3.01	3.05	
	psychological distress	4.28	4.38	4.58	4.59	4.65	4.49	
6 Baccalaureate	physical pain	3.19	3.28	3.24	3.26	3.09	3.35	
	psychological distress	4.15	4.26	4.55	4.50	4.44	4.72	
Graduate	physical pain							3.03
	psychological distress							4.54

manifested by students in the respective schools. Therefore, although the statistical analysis of the data revealed significant differences among schools, the exploration of variables that might have accounted for these differences did not suggest fruitful leads for further investigation.

Psychological distress. A two-way analysis of variance, with schools and time as the independent variables, was computed. Mean ratings are summarized in Table 12-1. The main effect for schools was not statistically significant but the main effect for time was significant beyond .001. The interaction between schools and time was also statistically significant beyond .001.

Inspection of Table 12-1 indicates that students in all six schools (with the possible exception of those in School 4) showed a similar pattern of change from entrance to graduation. That is, graduating students inferred considerably more psychological distress than did entering students. However, the schools did differ somewhat in the stage at which major differences in ratings were observed. For Schools 1, 2, 4, 5, and 6 the major difference was between the first year and the second year; for School 3 the major difference was between the fall and the spring of the first year.

It is of interest to note that students in School 3 entered with the highest ratings of pain and the lowest ratings of psychological distress. By the end of the first year, however, a large shift was noted along both dimensions. Their ratings of pain decreased markedly and their ratings of psychological distress increased markedly. Thus, their first year of nursing education clearly had a major impact on their beliefs about suffering. Nevertheless, a consideration of the curriculum of this school did not reveal any major differences, either in content or emphasis, from the other five schools studied.

Discussion

The principal finding of this research is that nursing education has a significant impact on students' beliefs about patients' suffering. Their beliefs about physical pain and psychological distress change in opposite directions. Specifically, their inferences of the amount of physical pain experienced by patients decrease and their inferences of the amount of psychological stress increase. Moreover, these changes appear to occur within the first year of nursing education.

Several factors might have accounted for these observed changes. Among the most important was the process of becoming "acculturated" within the subculture of nursing. A central aspect of this process undoubtedly involved acquiring the belief system shared by nurses, and one aspect of this belief system concerned patient suffering. As a result of day to day contact with nursing faculty, clinical supervisors, and graduate nurses, students were exposed to the beliefs that these nurses hold in common, and acquired these beliefs both as a result of direct instruction as well as identification with nursing models. As a senior nursing student in a baccalaureate program said during her interview:

> I've learned a lot about patients' suffering because of my instructors. They've not only been good role models as teachers but also as human beings. The way they talk to patients has shown me that a concern for people can be a very fulfilling part of life. Because of them I've decided to go on with my education.

Another student said:

> I know that the clinical instructors I have really have made a difference. Some are really into their profession, and help you understand how to work with patients. The instructors do a lot for helping you to put things into perspective.

Another factor, of course, was simply repeated exposure to patients who were suffering and the expectation that the student would respond as a professional. In our interviews with students, initial fear and anxiety were frequently mentioned in describing their early experiences with suffering patients, and the gradual reduction in this emotional reaction was interpreted in terms of becoming more objective and more professional. One student reported:

> I've gained more control with experience; in the beginning I was scared. Experience has been the best teacher. I don't feel helpless. I can find ways to help.

Another student said:

> I've learned to be more objective. I don't have to run to the nurse for an injection to give to the patient. At first I was frightened, but as I've gained more knowledge and understanding I realize pain can be psychological; for example, when you're sick and lonely it's far worse than for others.

Other students reported the following:

> I was pretty scared initially. Now I accept pain. Before I didn't have a reference point about patients' pain. I felt they all had a great deal of pain.

> I'm a lot more tolerant, able to curb my own anxieties so they don't interfere with my work.

> There was a time when I couldn't stand pain in others. I would feel like throwing up. Now I feel responsibility to act like a professional. I have more understanding of how to observe and how to behave.

> You learn to tolerate patient's pain. You accept it as something that has to be. I don't get as upset; I can observe pain more objectively. I used to worry about asking patients if they have pain; now I ask them questions and it doesn't bother me. As for myself, I'm more tolerant about my own pain.

> I'm not scared anymore. I'm much more objective. Patient pain is a problem but not mystical anymore. When I first was a student the pain seemed mysterious, unknown—that has changed. I'm a lot more tolerant of pain in people, and I've noticed that I've even become more tolerant of pain in myself.

> In the beginning I think all of us were caught up in ourselves—frightened

by the pain maybe, but now with experience and confidence pain isn't scary. Because the pain seemed to be everything I know I didn't look at the patient's other needs. Now I'm aware of the patient and the psychological needs. I can recognize when there's a psychological problem maybe making the pain worse.

You have to turn off the pain, otherwise you can't work. You have to learn to be objective. Nurses must learn control.

I've learned to set priorities. I'm more realistic. Sometimes there's only so much you can do about patient's pain.

Thus, as a result of their nursing education, these students learned that they could do something about patient's pain and discomfort (administer medication, change patients' position, and so on). Perhaps as a consequence of experience with these pain relieving procedures, their beliefs about patients' pain changed. After all, if a patient was experiencing pain, a nurse could take various steps to reduce the pain; therefore, when asked to evaluate the pain experienced by patients with various illnesses or injuries, the students with some clinical experience may very well have based their ratings on observations of patients whose pain had been relieved by appropriate nursing care. Therefore, this might have accounted for the reduced inferences of amount of pain characteristic of students beyond the first year of training.

In contrast to the decrease in pain ratings was the consistent increase in amount of psychological distress inferred by students after their initial year of training. This finding is highly congruent with our examination of the curricula in all six schools and the interview reports of the students. In every school, the psychological aspects of illness and injury were emphasized both in academic course work and in clinical supervision. This emphasis obviously had a major impact on students' beliefs. Among the numerous comments made about psychological distress, the following are a representative sample:

A lot of pain is fear I've learned so it's very important to understand a patient. I know with children they may not be as much in pain as scared and this makes the pain worse. You can do a lot by understanding the patient, and that's where psychology is so important. For example, a patient going up for surgery might have pain but much of the pain might also be anxiety and talking to the patient and preparing them for surgery can help reduce the pain.

The most important courses for me have been communication courses and my psych. courses, including psychopathology.

The psychological aspects of illness and pain have been stressed over and over again. Our program is geared to a holistic approach to nursing.

My courses and my instructors have made me a lot more aware of psychological aspects of suffering. I can accept the pain but I think I'm more aware of what people are feeling.

The whole first semester is devoted to how much patients need your attention. We have film strips, conferences and communication skills. A lot of stress is placed on psychology and sociology. I think we just realize how important the psychological aspects of a patient are.

No matter if there isn't much pain there's always some psychological distress in patients. I think we have to listen, ask questions, assess each situation. It depends on the patient, too; older people are lonely and there's a lot more psychological distress involved.

I can remember crying with a dying person. I cried because I felt helpless. Now I'm less emotional. I do what I can. Now I can say to her, 'it's sad,' and offer support.

The program has conditioned me to think about patients' psychological distress. As I get more experience I understand more about the psychological aspects of illness.

I'm aware that people can tolerate pain differently. I realize now you can't help some patients' pain. Sometimes the best thing to do is just stay with the patient. The pain is relieved psychologically.

I'm much more aware of psychological aspects. Before I started nursing school, I was kind and compassionate but now I have so much more understanding of what goes on with patients.

I've gained understanding that pain is a warning. I think that physical pain is a lot psychological. I know if you talk to a patient before you do a procedure they have less pain. My course work and my experience have made me more aware.

Examination of the curricula of the six schools studied, the reports of the students interviewed, and the changes in ratings of psychological distress over the course of training, clearly demonstrated the enormous impact of both academic and clinical experiences on nursing students' beliefs about suffering. As a consequence of their education, nursing students were sensitized to the psychological dimension of suffering, and indeed, consistently inferred greater psychological distress than physical pain in evaluating the experiences of patients with a variety of illnesses and injuries.

Implications for Nursing Education and Practice

The results of this research suggest that, while nursing education is highly successful in sensitizing prospective nurses to the psychological distress of patients, it may at the same time *desensitize* students to patients' pain. During the past decade or so in nursing education there has been a great deal of effort devoted to increasing nurses' awareness of psychological factors involved in nursing care. Our findings indicate that, to a large extent, these efforts have succeeded insofar as nursing students' sensitivity to psychological distress is concerned. However, two problems suggest themselves in this context.

Having sensitized students to patients' psychological distress, it is not at all clear that nursing education also prepares nurses to deal effectively with this distress within the limitations confronted by most nurses in actual hospital practice. Given the demands of typical hospital environments, the time-consuming and emotionally demanding psychotherapeutically based techniques of dealing with psychological distress are often not practical, and sometimes not even possible. During training, with limited responsibilities and duties, nursing students may well have the opportunity to engage in extended conversations with their patients, gain empathic understanding, and provide psychological support. But in actual nursing practice, these opportunities are likely to be severely limited. Our observations of nurse-patient interactions reported in a preceding chapter indicate that the great majority of these interactions are very brief. Obviously, this is not a function of the nurses' insensitivity to patients' psychological distress; our research clearly points in exactly the opposite direction. By and large, nurses are in fact very sensitive to the psychological dimensions of suffering. But given the exigencies of practice in most hospital situations, there is little opportunity to use techniques effectively that demand a considerable amount of uninterrupted time and a good deal of energy. As a result, nurses who have been sensitized to patients' psychological distress may very well feel frustrated and patients experiencing this distress may not receive the care which reduces this aspect of their suffering.

Thus, nursing education has successfully solved part of this general problem: nursing students are being sensitized to the psychological dimension of patient suffering. But the second part of this problem involves the development of nursing techniques and procedures that effectively relieve patient distress and are practically feasible within the actual conditions of typical hospital practice. This part of the problem remains unsolved, and it presents a major challenge for future nursing research.

A second issue concerns the significant reduction in amount of pain inferred by students as a consequence of their educational experiences. In a sense, student nurses are "taught" that patients feel less pain than these students believed patients did upon entering training. Perhaps this was an inevitable part of the process of what students during our interviews characterized as becoming "objective" or "professional." Indeed, it seemed reasonable to expect a certain degree of emotional distancing between nurse and patient in the course of a student's professional development. As the students in our sample indicated, this distancing was not only desirable, but also necessary in order to function effectively in providing nursing care.

There also may be some potential danger in this educational process. Too much desensitization to patient pain, too much emotional distance between nurse and patient, too much reliance on routine procedures for relieving pain may significantly decrease the quality of nursing care. The present study does not provide a specific guideline to evaluate nursing education in these terms; however, the results suggest that nursing educators may profitably devote some attention to what their students are learning about patients' experiences of pain as well as psychological distress.

Part Five
Beliefs and Behaviors

This section deals with the central problem of the relation between nurses' beliefs about suffering and their nursing behavior in actual interactions with patients. Three interrelated studies are reported. The first deals with nurses in medical-surgical units, the second concerns nurses in obstetric units, and the third focuses on nurses in pediatric units. Thus, the relation between nurses' beliefs and their nursing behavior is considered in three different nursing settings.

13

Inferences of Suffering and Nursing Behaviors Among Medical-Surgical, Obstetric, and Pediatric Nurses

The preceding studies have focused on nurses' reactions to suffering and have identified a number of variables that influence these inferences. From a theoretical point of view, these previous investigations have been extremely productive in clarifying nurses' reactions to the pain and psychological distress experienced by patients. In practical terms, however, the pragmatic value of studying nurses' reactions to suffering depends, to a large extent, on the demonstrable relation between these reactions and actual nursing behavior. The present research, therefore, was undertaken to investigate this relationship.

We began this research with the assumption that most students who entered nursing training were especially sensitive to the pain and distress of others. The desire to alleviate suffering was probably a major source of motivation leading to the choice of a nursing career. But over the course of training and practice, as a result of the personal discomfort experienced while working closely with suffering patients, some nurses developed mechanisms that helped maintain psychological distance between themselves and their patients' suffering. If this distance was not achieved, working day to day with people in pain and psychological distress would probably have become intolerable, and the person would have been likely to escape from the situation, either by leaving nursing or by seeking nursing activities other than the direct care of patients.

One way to achieve this kind of psychological distance is to minimize the pain and distress inferred about patients; that is, caring for suffering patients becomes psychologically safer or more tolerable if the nurse can believe that the patient "is really not suffering too much." Thus, nurses' inferences of relatively low suffering among patients may be viewed, in part, as a defensive or distancing mechanism that permits the nurse to maintain her own psychological integrity in the face of daily contact with people in pain, people who are experiencing considerable psychological distress, and people who may be dying.

The tendency to achieve some psychological distance by minimizing the patient's suffering may be reinforced by cultural factors, such that nurses who come from cultural backgrounds that prize relatively stoic, emotionally nonexpressive attitudes may be more likely to use this mechanism in their professional adjustment. In contrast, nurses from cultural backgrounds that are characteristically more expressive may be less likely to adapt to the stresses of nursing by minimizing patients' suffering, though presumably they use other means of dealing with this psychological issue. This general expectation is supported by our previous finding that nurses from northern European family backgrounds tend to infer less suffering than do nurses from southern European backgrounds, assuming that the stereotype of the emotionally expressive Mediterranean in contrast to the more stoic Anglo-Saxon/Germanic or Scandinavian reflects broad cultural differences.

In any event, if low inferences of suffering represent, at least in part, a defensive mechanism some nurses use to make their daily contact with pain and distress psychologically tolerable, it would be reasonable to expect similar distancing in nursing behavior. Thus, comparing nurses who infer high degrees of suffering with those who infer relatively lower degrees of suffering, one would expect the high inference group to be emotionally more supportive of the patient, more concerned with interpersonal and comforting aspects of nursing care, and psychologically closer to the patient as manifested in the emotional tone of communications and physical contact with the patient. On the other hand, the low inference group would be expected to evince more interest in technical aspects of nursing, be less supportive of patients' complaints, and be more distant both emotionally and in terms of physical contact with patients.

To investigate the relation between inferences of suffering and nursing behaviors, a series of three studies was conducted to compare the behaviors of nurses who inferred high patient suffering versus those who inferred relatively low patient suffering. The first study considered nurses working in medical-surgical units, the second study focused on nurses in obstetric units, and the third study involved nurses in pediatric units. Thus, the relation between inferences of suffering and nursing behavior could be evaluated in three different nursing settings.

Study One: Medical-Surgical Nurses

Subjects

Using the *Standard Measure of Inferences of Suffering,* data were obtained from 272 nurses in four large metropolitan hospitals. All of these nurses were currently assigned to the medical-surgical unit of their respective hospitals, and all volunteered to serve as subjects of this research. Each *S* received a total inferred suffering score, which was the average rating of pain and psychological distress over all items. Inferred suffering score could range from 2 to 14. In the present sample, the range of scores extended from 2.30 to 4.91.

To select high inference and low inference groups, the 27 nurses (10 percent of the sample) who received the largest total inferred suffering scores and the 27 nurses who received the smallest scores were identified. For this sample, the tenth percentile was 3.05, and the ninetieth percentile was 4.45; thus, the low inference group had total inferred suffering scores of 3.05 or lower, while the high inference group had scores of 4.45 or higher.

The 54 nurses in these two groups were contacted and told that the next step in the research involved observations of their nursing interactions with patients. All 54 nurses volunteered to participate; however, because of scheduling problems, complete data could be obtained for only 26 nurses in the high inference group and 23 nurses in the low inference group.

Observations of nursing behaviors. On the basis of a review of relevant literature, a first draft of an observation schedule to record nursing behaviors was developed. In the course of several meetings with over 25 currently practicing nurses on medical-surgical units, numerous suggestions were obtained regarding additions to and revisions of this initial schedule. The revised schedule was tried out in observations of six nurses, and, on the basis of this experience, a final form of the observation schedule was constructed.

In developing this schedule, several aims were kept in mind. First, the schedule had to provide an objective basis for obtaining reliable observations. Second, the method of recording data had to be concise and rapid enough to be useful in collecting observations that sometimes involved a series of quickly occurring events. Third, the method of observing and recording had to be as unobtrusive as possible, with little or no disruption of the ongoing nurse-patient interaction. Fourth, the schedule had to provide a basis for recording the range of nurse behavior in relation to patients likely to be in a medical-surgical setting.

The schedule is composed of three major sections. The first section deals with the nurses' verbal behavior, and includes categories such as the following: asks an opening question, dismisses patient's worries or concerns, gives an order or directive, and replies to patient's questions. A total of 14 categories are in this section, and the observer is required to merely check those categories that apply to the nurse's verbal behavior, with a brief note concerning questions about coding. In those few instances when the observer is not immediately sure of the appropriate category, the notes are reviewed by two researchers, and the statement classified.

The second section of the observation schedule concerns nursing actions. These include, for example: backrub, changes dressings, gives medication, straightens bedding, fixtures, and so on. A total of 14 categories are included in this section.

The third section covers the nurses' relation to the patient. For each interaction, the observer makes ratings on a three-point scale (low, medium, high) for six dimensions of the nurse's behavior: physical distance, emotional tone, level of activity, attention to patient, touching, and gentleness. Each point on the three-point rating scale for each dimension is defined. For example, the three points for the dimension of Physical Distance are defined as follows: *low* means that the nurse is far away from the patient, for example, if the patient is in bed, the nurse stands near the door of the room; if the patient is in the hall, the nurse remains at the nursing station, behind the desk; *medium* means that the nurse stands somewhat near the patient, but not within touching distance, for example, if the patient is in bed, the nurse stands near the foot of the bed; *high* means that the nurse stands very close to the patient, for example, if the patient is in bed, the nurse stands next to the head of the bed near the patient's head; patient and nurse are within touching distance of each other.

Ratings for *Emotional Tone* are defined as follows: *low* involves an emotional tone that may be characterized as hostile, irritated, cold, or withdrawn; *medium* involves an emotional tone that may be characterized as neutral, business-like, matter of fact; *high* involves an emotional tone that may be characterized as very warm and pleasant.

A summary of the categories contained in the observation schedule is presented in Table 13-1. Brief definitions are included for each category under verbal interactions and nurse's relation to patient; it is assumed that the meaning of each category under nursing actions is self-evident.

Procedure

Observations were made only during the daytime shift on the medical-surgical unit of each hospital. On a given day, an observer was assigned to accompany one nurse who was either in the high inference or low inference group. The observer, of course, did not know which group the nurse was in. Each observer, a nurse, wore her regular nursing uniform. However, in the course of the observations, the observer did not participate at all in the nurse-patient interactions. In fact, the observer made every effort to "fade into the background" of the nurse-patient interactions, and reports from both participating nurses and observers indicated that this was successfully achieved. Before observations were started on a particular unit, patients were informed that some of the nurses on the unit would occasionally be accompanied by a nurse-observer who was interested in the nursing that went on in the unit but would not participate in the process of nursing care. Patients accepted this explanation and observers had no interaction with patients. Nurses who were subjects in this study indicated that, at first, they were conscious of the

Figure 13–1
Observational Categories for Study of Medical-Surgical Nurses

---

Nurse's Verbal Interaction with Patient

---

1. *Asks an opening question.* Nurse asks patient a direct question. For example: What is wrong? Where does it hurt? Why did you call? Briefly note the nature of the question.

2. *Changes subject; brings up another topic.* During any part of interaction nurse switches the subject from the patient's problem or complaint. For example: talks about weather, asks patient about family, general chatting about any other subject other than the issue of the interaction.

3. *Chats about condition.* Talks about patient's condition in a general way. For example: Let's see what's going on. Now here, let's take a look and see what is what.

4. *Defends actions or behaviors, for example, offers excuses or apologies.* Nurse defends actions. For example: Someone always comes as soon as you call. We're very busy on the floor now. We have to do it this way. We know it isn't easy but this has to be done.

5. *Dismisses patient's worries or concerns.* For example: Your stitches aren't that bad. There's a patient we had in last week who had twice as many.

6. *Doesn't say anything.* Nurse is silent.

7. *Explains, teaches, gives information.*

8. *Explores patient's feelings.*
   a. *Physical.* Can you tell me where it hurts? What is the pain like?
   b. *Psychological.* Can you tell me what is bothering you? Is something on your mind?

9. *Gives an order or directive.* Specifically tells patient to do something. For example: Take the medicine now. Open your mouth. Turn over on your stomach.

10. *Referrals.* Nurse calls another individual in to patient or sends another individual in to patient.

11. *Replies to patient's questions.* Patient asks a question and nurse gives a direct answer. For example: Patient: Please give me something for my headache. Nurse: I'll get you something for your pain. Patient: Can you do anything about the light? Nurse: I'll draw the curtains around your bed.

12. *Sympathetic understanding/reassurance.* For example: I know just how you feel. I know it isn't comfortable now, but it won't be long.

13. *Verbalizes nursing action to be taken.* For example: I'm going to just put the injection here; first, I'm going to have you hold your hand here. It will just take a second.

14. *Other.* Any other verbalization should be briefly noted.

(continued)

Figure 13-1 continued

Nursing Actions

---

1. *Backrub*
2. *Catheterization*
3. *Changes dressings*
4. *Changes patient's position*
5. *Checks instruments*
6. *Demonstrates technique*
7. *Fixes I.V.*
8. *Gives medication*
9. *Informs doctor of patient's condition*
10. *Physical nurturing, for example, gives blanket, turns on TV, gives tray*
11. *Refers patient to another staff member*
12. *Straightens bedding, fixtures, and so on*
13. *Teaches or demonstrates*
14. *Other (specify)*

Nurse's Relation to Patient

---

1. *Physical Distance.* This refers to how near the nurse is to patient.
   Low: Nurse is far away from patient. Stands near door. Remains at nurse's station behind desk and talks to patient in hall.
   Medium: Nurse stands somewhat near patient. For example: patient is in bed and nurse stands near foot of bed.
   High: Nurse stands very close to patient. If patient is in bed, nurse stands next to the head of bed near patient's head. Patient and nurse are within "touching" distance of each other.

2. *Emotional Tone.* This refers to the overall emotional style of the nurse. Facial expression, voice, gestures, words.
   Low: Hostile, irritated, cold, withdrawn.
   Medium: Neutral, businesslike, matter-of-fact.
   High: Very warm, smiles a great deal, pleasant.

3. *Level of Activity.* Refers to nurse's physical movements: how she walks, arm and hand movements, and so on.
   Low: Nurse walks slowly. Actions are deliberate. Hands move slowly. Body quiet.
   Medium: Walks and moves at a normal rate.
   High: Nurse moves very quickly. Walks at a fast pace. Hands move quickly. A great deal of activity.

4. *Attention to Patient.*
   Low: Nurse looks away from patient, appears distracted. For example: talks to patient and at the same time is carrying on a conversation with another person, backs off from patient quickly, moves toward door or away from patient's bed or patient.

Medium: Nurse looks at patient. Appears to listen and to react.
High: Nurse is very attentive. Leans towards patient; concentrates on patient. No attempt to leave quickly. Eyes directed toward patient the whole time of interaction. Doesn't look away.

5 . *Touching.*
Low: Nurse does not touch patient except to perform a technique. No placing or laying on of hands.
Medium: Slight touching of patient.
High: A great deal of touching of patient. Pats patient's hand, places arm around patient, holds patient's hand while talking. Touches patient a great deal.

6 . *Gentleness*
Low: Rough, hard.
Medium: Neither rough nor gentle.
High: Especially gentle, soft.

---

observer and felt the observer's presence might have affected their behavior. However, they also reported that after a very short time, as they became involved in their work, they behaved as they usually did and felt the observer had little or no influence on what they did. It was impossible, of course, to evaluate objectively, the effect of the observer's presence, but our evidence at least suggested that the observer's efforts to "fade into the background" were generally successful, and while one would assume the observers had some effect, it seems reasonable to suggest that this effect was minimized. Moreover, there was no evidence to indicate a differential effect on nurses in the high inference or low inference groups, and it may therefore be assumed that, whatever minimal effect the presence of observers might have had, it did not systematically bias the crucial comparisons between nurses in the two groups.

An observer accompanied each nurse for an entire morning or afternoon, recording all nurse-patient interactions that explicitly involved physical pain, discomfort, or psychological distress of the patient. Obviously, in the course of routine nursing care, many nurse-patient interactions were not concerned directly with patient suffering. Although of general interest in studying nursing behavior, those interactions not concerned with patient suffering were not the focus of this research and were therefore not recorded. Thus, the data dealt only with nurse-patient interactions that were immediately concerned with one or another aspect of a patient's suffering.

Reliability of Observations and Data Analysis

Two observers were used in the final data collection. Both were graduate nurses with over eight years of hospital nursing experience, and both were currently enrolled in advanced degree programs in nursing. The first step in training the observers involved careful discussion of the code book, clarifying each of the categories contained in the observational schedule. This was followed by practice observations of actual nurse-patient interactions, followed by further discussion of the various categories in the schedule and the observers' responses. Finally, to evaluate reliability of the observations, both observers recorded the behavior of five nurses in interaction with patients on their units. A total of 42 interactions were recorded by both observers, and reliability was evaluated by computing percentage of agreement for each of the major sections of the observation schedule. For nurse's verbal behavior, agreement was 88 percent; for nursing actions, agreement was 90 percent; and for nurse's relation to patient, agreement was 83 percent. Thus, for both verbal behavior and nursing actions the reliability of observations was high. As might be expected, agreement on the several dimensions of the nurse's relation to patient was somewhat lower, but clearly acceptable for the purposes of this research.

For each nurse the final scores used in the data analysis were based on observations of five nurse-patient interactions explicitly involving patient suffering. In the course of the data collections, many more interactions were recorded for most nurses. However, the minimum number recorded for any one nurse during the observation period was five. Therefore, rather than introduce a possible bias by basing final scores for nursing behavior on varying numbers of interactions for different nurses, scores for each nurse in the sample were based on the first five interactions recorded for that nurse. It should be noted that in a preliminary investigation conducted prior to data collection for the main study, the results indicated that five interactions provided a minimum base for obtaining a relatively stable description of the pattern of a nurse's behavior. Frequencies in particular categories varied, of course, with additional observations, but the nurse's overall pattern of behavior appeared to remain rather stable.

For each category of verbal behaviors and nursing actions, each nurse received a score representing the number of times the particular behavior was exhibited. Thus, for example, if a nurse asked an opening question in three interactions, he or she received a score of three for that category. Similarly, if a nurse gave medications during two interactions, a score of two was received for that category of nursing action. For the six dimensions of nurse's relation to patient, the average rating for each dimension served as the score of that dimension. To evaluate the differences between mean scores for the nurses in the high inference and low inference groups, *t* tests were computed and the null hypothesis rejected at the .05 level.

Results

Verbal interactions. The most frequent category of behavior was "Asks opening question" (mean score 3.77), followed by "Gives order" (2.53), and "Verbalizes, explains actions to be taken" (2.45). Somewhat less frequent were "Replies to patient's question" (1.84), "Sympathetic understanding, reassurance" (1.31), and "Explains, gives information" (1.04). All of the other categories of verbal behavior were considerably less frequent, having occurred, on the average, less than once. Thus, in interactions involving patient pain or psychological distress, the nurse typically asked the patient what was wrong, told the patient what to do, and explained some nursing action about to be taken. In contrast, there was relatively little general discussion of the patient's condition and very little exploration of the patient's feelings. From the point of view of verbal interactions, it seemed likely that the nurse's primary focus was on the patient's immediate complaint and on actions taken in direct response to this complaint.

Nursing actions. Most frequent actions taken by nurses in this sample were some form of physical nurturing (mean score 0.90) and the closely related category of changing the patient's position (0.69). Perhaps more noteworthy than the relative frequencies of various categories were the generally low frequencies across all categories. No single category of nursing action occurred with an average frequency greater than one, suggesting that the majority of nurse-patient interactions involved verbal exchanges rather than specific non-verbal nursing actions.

Differences between High and Low Inference Groups

Verbal interactions. Although 13 different categories of verbal behavior were observed, not all of these categories were relevant to the expected differences between the high and low inference groups. In the absence of previous research dealing with the relation between reactions to suffering and nursing behavior, it was difficult to formulate hypotheses about specific behaviors. However, it was generally expected that nurses who tended to infer relatively high levels of suffering would be more concerned about patients' feelings and less likely to distance themselves from their patients or attempt to block expressions of feeling. One cannot measure these expectations directly, but in terms of the specific categories of verbal behavior observed, it seemed reasonable to expect the high inference group to show more frequent behavior in the following categories of verbal interaction: (1) chats about condition, (2) defends, explains action; (3) explains, gives information; (4) explores feelings, (5) sympathetic understanding, reassurances; and (6) verbalizes, explains actions to be taken. Each of these categories reflects, either directly or indirectly, active concern with the patient's point of view and thus seemed to be congruent with a tendency to pay attention to the patient's feelings. In contrast, one would have expected the high inference group less frequently to change the subject when a patient complained or to dismiss the patient's concerns.

At the outset of this research we did not consider these expectations to be formal hypotheses; rather, they served as a guide for our exploration of this area of research and a basis for our data analysis. Thus, our findings with respect to these particular categories of behavior cannot be interpreted as firm conclusions, but must be viewed as promising leads for further research.

The comparisons of verbal interactions showed statistically significant differences for three of the eight relevant categories. Specifically, the high inference group more frequently explained to patients past or future nursing actions (significant beyond .02) and less frequently dismissed their patients' concerns (significant beyond .05). No significant differences were obtained for: (1) changes subject, (2) chats about condition, (3) explains, gives information; (4) explores feelings, and (5) sympathetic understanding, reassurance. It should be noted that there were no significant differences between the two groups of nurses for the five categories not relevant to our initial expectations.

Nursing actions. Just as we could not formulate with confidence formal hypotheses regarding particular verbal behaviors, we could not make firm predictions about specific nursing actions. Nevertheless, on the basis of our speculations about the underlying psychological meaning of the tendency to infer either relatively high or low suffering, we expected certain differences in nursing actions. In general, we expected high inference nurses to behave in ways that reflected greater concern with patient comfort, while low inference nurses were expected to show more frequent behavior in categories unrelated to the patient's feelings. Specifically, the high inference group was expected to have higher scores in three categories: (1) backrub, (2) changes patient's position, and (3) physical nurturing. The low inference group was expected to have higher scores in: (1) checks instruments, and (2) straightens bedding, and so on.

Several categories of nursing action involved more or less common nursing behaviors that seemed unlikely to be related to a nurse's tendency to infer either high or low levels of suffering. For example, the decision to change a patient's dressing was most likely to depend upon a particular routine of nursing care or the observation of a physical sign indicating the need to change a dressing, and while a nurse's inference about a patient's feeling might have played some role in this decision, it seemed unlikely to be a major factor in most instances of this nursing action. Similarly, one would not have expected a nurse's inferences of suffering to be consistently related to: (1) catheterization, (2) demonstrates technique, (3) adjusts I.V., (4) gives medication, (5) informs doctor, or (6) teaches. Nursing actions in all of these categories, of course, might very well have been influenced by a nurse's judgments about a patient's feelings, but the influence of other determinants, such as the routines of nursing care or the observation of a physical sign, would have been likely to obviate any relationship between inferences of suffering and these particular behaviors.

Comparisons of nursing actions showed, as expected, that nurses in the high inference group more frequently changed their patients' positions (significant beyond .05) and less frequently engaged in "straightening" behaviors (.05). However, no significant differences were obtained for: (1) backrub, (2) checks instruments, or (3) physical nurturing. The high and low inference groups did not differ significantly in any of the nonrelevant categories.

Relation to patient. In addition to categorizing the nurse's specific behaviors, observers also related the overall nurse-patient relationship for each interaction. These ratings were made along six dimensions, four of which were relevant to the expectations of this study. Specifically, nurses in the high inference group were expected to stand closer to patients, convey a warmer emotional tone, touch the patient more frequently, and be more gentle in their interactions. Accordingly, these expectations would be reflected by higher ratings in the physical distance, emotional tone, touching, and gentleness scales. Although the nurse's level of activity and degree of attention to patient were also rated, neither of these scales was relevant to our initial expectations. In interpreting these results it should be recalled that, as noted earlier, the observers who made these ratings did not know whether the nurse they were rating at any given time was in the high or low inference group.

Ratings of the nurses' relation to patients indicated that three of our four expectations in this area were fulfilled: high inference nurses tended to stand closer to their patients, conveyed a warmer emotional tone, and touched their patients more often (all significant beyond .05). There was no significant difference in degree of gentleness and neither of the two nonrelevant scales showed a reliable difference.

Discussion

At the outset of this study we could not, with confidence, make precise predictions about how nurses' beliefs would be related to specific nursing behaviors. However, at a more general level, we expected nurses who tended to infer high suffering to behave differently from nurses who tended to infer low suffering. On the basis of speculations that interpreted inferences of low suffering primarily as part of a defensive system designed to reduce the amount of stress experienced by a nurse during everyday contact with the suffering of others, we expected the low inference group to display parallel patient-distancing behavior in actual interactions with patients. That was precisely the nature of the results obtained. In fact, low inference nurses actually tended to stand further away from patients than did high inference nurses; thus, physical distance seemed to mirror the psychological distance between nurse and patient.

In addition to greater physical distance from the patient, the nurse who inferred relatively low suffering also tended to be emotionally more neutral or matter of fact vis-a-vis the patient, touched the patient less frequently, engaged in somewhat more impersonal nursing actions, tended to dismiss patients' worries more frequently, and less often discussed or explained nursing actions. In general, then, nurses in the low inference group, in comparison to those in the high inference group, were more impersonal and distant in their interactions with patients. In short, their behavior reflected and mirrored their beliefs about patient suffering.

Although the results of this study provided evidence that nurses' beliefs about suffering were related to their nursing behavior, care must be taken in generalizing these results. First, it should be noted that this study was designed primarily as exploratory research, and although we were able to evaluate certain expectations in terms of data obtained, we did not test specific predictions of formal hypotheses. In fact, we viewed the research as an empirical basis for formulating such hypotheses.

Second, it is important to note that all of our expectations were supported. For verbal interactions, three of eight expected differences were statistically significant; for nursing actions, two of the five expected differences were statistically significant; and for ratings concerning nurse-patient relation, three of four expected differences were statistically significant. In no case, were the obtained differences significant in the direction opposite to our expectations. Therefore, while the overall results clearly supported the general proposition that nurses' beliefs about patient suffering were related to their actual nursing behavior, at this point in the line of investigation we could not with confidence specify the relation between beliefs about suffering and particular nursing behavior.

Finally, it must be noted that all of the nurses observed in this study were working in medical-surgical units. In other settings, working with different kinds of patients and engaged in somewhat different kinds of nursing tasks, the relation between beliefs and behavior may have differed from that found for medical-surgical nurses. Thus, the results of this initial study relating beliefs to behavior were clearly encouraging, but firm conclusions in this area of research must await further investigation.

Study Two: Obstetric Nurses

The aim of our second study in this particular line of research was to determine whether nurses' beliefs about suffering and nursing behaviors were related in a setting quite different from the usual medical-surgical unit. Of the many possibilities available, the obstetrics unit was chosen as one which was clearly different in many respects from the medical-surgical unit. It also provided a setting in which nurses had to frequently deal with the issue of patients' pain.

Our general expectation was essentially the same as that underlying the initial study of medical-surgical nurses. That is, the tendency to infer relatively low suffering in patients was viewed primarily as a defensive mechanism which would be reflected by nursing behaviors that increased the psychological distance between nurse and patient. Because of the difference in settings and in the kinds of demands made upon the nurse, we did not expect the results for obstetric nurses to be identical to those obtained for medical-surgical nurses. Nevertheless, the direction of differences between obstetric nurses who inferred relatively high patient suffering versus those who inferred low patient suffering was expected to be essentially similar to the differences obtained in the preceding study.

Method

The design of this study replicated that of the initial study of medical-surgical nurses. From a large sample of obstetric nurses, a group who tended to infer relatively high patient suffering and a group who tended to infer relatively low patient suffering were identified. Nurse-patient interactions of nurses in these two groups were observed and their behaviors compared in terms of verbal interactions, nursing actions, and relation to patient.

Subjects

One hundred and thirty eight obstetric nurses in 14 hospitals in the New York-New Jersey area comprised the initial sample. Using the *Standard Measure of Inferences of Suffering,* scores were obtained for the entire sample. The total inferred suffering score, which was the average rating of pain and psychological distress over all items, served as the basis for identifying the high and low inference groups. The high inference group was composed of the 25 nurses with the highest total score (scores $\leq$ 4.26) and the low inference group was composed of the 25 nurses with the lowest total score (scores $\leq$ 3.29). The two groups did not differ significantly in age, years of nursing, educational background, or in work shift.

Procedure

As in the preceding study a nurse-observer accompanying each nurse in the sample observed and recorded the nurse's interactions with patients. To account for the somewhat different actions taken by obstetric nurses in comparison to those in the medical-surgical unit, the observation schedule was slightly revised. "Administering an enema" was added to the category including catheterization; "teaches and demonstrates techniques" were combined in a single category; and the following categories were added to the list under nursing actions: (1) listens to fetal heart; (2) palpates abdomen, times contractions; (3) checks bladder, breasts, uterus, perineum; (4) touching, holding, cuddling, stroking; (5) T.P.R., blood pressure; and (6) checks supplies. In all other respects the procedure followed in this study replicated that described in the study of medical-surgical nurses.

To increase reliability of measurement, 10 interactions (rather than five as in the previous study) were observed and recorded. Reliability of observations was evaluated by comparing the two observer's ratings of 30 nurse-patient interactions, and agreement of over 90 percent was obtained for all categories.

Results

Verbal interactions. The most frequent category of verbal interactions was "explains, gives information," which occurred, on the average, in nearly 70 percent of the nurse-patient interactions observed (mean score 6.86). This was followed closely by "explores feelings" (5.61) and "gives orders" (5.50), both of which occurred in nearly 60 percent of the interactions. "Sympathetic understanding, reassurance" (4.63), and "verbalizes, explains actions to be taken" (4.49), were next most frequent, with a sharp drop in frequency for all other verbal behavior.

The observed differences in verbal behavior between obstetric and medical-surgical nurses obviously reflected the differences between the two nursing situations. Among medical-surgical nurses the most frequent verbal behavior was "asks opening question," which usually initiated an interaction. In the medical-surgical unit a patient feeling some distress typically called for a nurse, and in responding, the nurse's first step would have been to find out why the patient called. In this setting there was a wide range of reasons that might have accounted for a patient's call, and the nurse's initial inquiry was clearly an important first step in most interactions. For the obstetric nurse the range of likely problems was much more restricted and contact with the patient did not nearly as often depend upon a patient's call. Thus, asking an opening question did not occur as often because the nurse was, in most instances, already aware of the situation to be confronted in most interactions.

Giving information and giving orders were high frequency behaviors for both obstetric and medical-surgical nurses, but "explores feelings" was much more frequent for the obstetric nurse. Once again, this clearly reflected the differences in nursing situations; the obstetric nurse's actions depended, to a certain extent, on the patient's subjective report of her experiences, and thus the nurse frequently looked for this information from the patient.

It should be noted also that sympathetic understanding and reassurance were expressed much more often by the obstetric nurse (in approximately 46 percent of the interactions observed) than by the medical-surgical nurse (in approximately 26 percent of interactions). This finding, too, reflected differences in the situations. In many instances obstetric patients were clearly and obviously experiencing pain and the nurse responded with understanding and reassurance. Among medical-surgical patients the pain or psychological distress might not have been so obvious and the expression of sympathetic understanding was less frequently elicited.

Nursing actions. The highest frequency category of nursing actions for this sample was "straightens bedding, and so on" (mean score 2.70), followed by "changes patient's position" (2.65), "checks bladder, breasts, uterus, perineum" (2.41), and "palpates abdomen, times contractions" (2.31). These latter categories obviously reflected the particular demands of the obstetric nursing situation.

Comparing frequencies obtained for nurses revealed the differences between these two nursing settings. For the obstetric nurse, six categories occurred on the average, in at least 20 percent of the interactions, while for the medical-surgical nurses no single category occurred as often as 20 percent of the time. Presumably, this reflects the heterogeneity of demands of medical-surgical nursing in contrast to obstetric nursing.

An unexpected finding was the relatively high frequency of various "straightening" behavior found among this sample of obstetric nurses (27 percent for obstetric nurses in comparison to approximately 12 percent for medical-surgical nurses). It was difficult to interpret this finding with much confidence, but perhaps some of the obstetric nurses' "straightening" behavior might have served as a tension-reducing mechanism for nurses working in a situation likely to be characterized by a relatively high degree of tension.

Differences between High and Low Inference Groups

Verbal interactions. Of the expected differences in comparisons of verbal interactions of nurses in the high and low inference groups only one was statistically significant; nurses in the high inference group more frequently expressed sympathetic understanding and reassurance to their patients (significant beyond .05). None of the other categories of verbal interaction, either relevant or nonrelevant to the expected differences, showed significant differences between the two groups of nurses.

Nursing actions. In comparing the high and low inference groups on nursing actions, only one category relevant to expected differences showed a statistically significant difference; nurses in the high inference group tended to touch their patients more frequently (significant beyond .05). None of the other categories, either relevant or nonrelevant, revealed significant results.

Relation to patient. None of the comparisons of the relation to patient for obstetric nurses revealed significant differences. It may be noted that under nursing actions, high inference nurses received significantly higher scores in the category dealing with touching the patient; in the ratings of relation to patient, however, the parallel dimension of "amount of touching" as a relation to patient did not reveal a significant difference. It seemed reasonable to view the observations under nursing actions as a somewhat more precise measure than the overall rating made under relations to patients. In the ratings, the results for the dimension dealing with amount of touching were in the expected direction, but perhaps the ratings were not sensitive enough to reveal the small, though statistically significant, differences shown in the analysis of nursing actions.

Discussion

Both of the statistically signficant differences obtained in this study were in the direction expected and were congruent with the general trend of results obtained for medical-surgical nurses. Nevertheless, nurses in the high inference and low inference groups did not differ reliably in any of the other categories observed. Thus, for obstetric nurses, the expected relation between beliefs and behavior was at best minimal, supported only by observations that high inference nurses more often expressed sympathetic understanding and reassurance and touched their patients somewhat more frequently.

The results of this study suggest that the relation between nurses' beliefs and their nursing behaviors is mediated by the situation in which the nursing occurs. In an obstetric setting, perhaps the immediate situational demands are so compelling that the effects of a nurse's belief about patients' experiences are obscured. For example, during a patient's labor, a nurse's actions are likely to be determined primarily by the observation of physical signs indicative of the progress of labor. It is generally assumed that the patient in labor will experience some pain and while evidence of very severe distress will undoubtedly influence a nurse's behavior, relatively small differences in the amount of suffering inferred probably play a minor role in determining the obstetric nurse's actions. In obstetric nursing, then, situational factors rather than a particular nurse's beliefs may be the predominant influence on behavior.

Study Three: Pediatric Nurses

Having studied the relation between nurses' beliefs about suffering and their nursing behaviors among medical-surgical and obstetric nurses this study was undertaken to investigate the same relationships in still another setting. There were, of course, a number of possibilities that might have been selected, but a primary consideration at this stage of the research was to focus on a patient population that was clearly different from those found in a medical-surgical or obstetric unit. In the preceding studies all of the patients were adults, and this factor itself may have had some influence on the relation between nurses' beliefs and behaviors. Therefore, to investigate the same general problem with a distinctly different group of patients, nurses working in pediatric units were chosen as the focus of the third study in this series.

Method

The design of this study replicated that of the preceding two studies, with the exception of the nature of the sample.

One hundred and thirty three nurses working in pediatric units of 13 hospitals in the New York-New Jersey area were tested with the *Standard Measure of Inferences of Suffering*. Using the average ratings of physical pain and psychological distress over all items, the 25 nurses scoring highest and the 25 nurses scoring lowest were identified. The high inference group had scores equal to or greater than 4.31; the low inference group had scores equal to or less than 3.15. The two groups did not differ significantly in age, years of nursing, educational background, or work shift.

Procedure

As in the preceding studies, a nurse-observer accompanying each nurse in the sample observed and recorded the nurses' reactions with patients. For the present study, one category, "adjusts language to patient" was added to the list of observed verbal interactions, and the three categories designed for the study of obstetric nursing (listens to fetal heart, and so on) were omitted. The results for each subject were based on data obtained from 10 nurse-patient interactions.

Results

Verbal interactions. By far the most frequent category of verbal interactions for this sample of pediatric nurses was "explores feelings," which occurred in over 50 percent of the interactions observed (mean score 5.34). "Explains, gives information" (3.75), and "gives orders" (3.73) were next highest in frequency, both having occurred in about 37 percent of the interactions. The next highest category was "chats about condition," with a frequency of 36 percent (3.60) with approximately the same percentage (35.5) found for "verbalizes, explains actions to be taken" (3.55).

In general, these results suggest that the pediatric nurses in this sample talked a good deal more with their patients than did the medical-surgical or obstetric nurses sampled in the preceding studies. Compare, for example, the results for pediatric and medical-surgical nurses in terms of two categories, "explores feelings" and "chats about condition." Both of these categories occurred in less than 10 percent of the interactions observed among medical-surgical nurses and their patients. In contrast, both of these categories had very high frequencies (53 percent and 36 percent, respectively) for pediatric nurses. It would seem, therefore, that pediatric nurses in comparison to medical-surgical nurses spend a good deal more time chatting with their patients and exploring their patients' feelings.

The differences between pediatric and obstetric nurses are less striking than those between pediatric and medical-surgical nurses. For both pediatric and obstetric nurses, exploring patients' feelings occurred in over 50 percent of the interactions observed. However, obstetric nurses much more frequently gave explanations and provided information to their patients (nearly 70 percent of interactions for obstetric nurses and less than 40 percent for pediatric nurses). It would seem likely that this difference reflected differences both in the nursing tasks and the patient populations in obstetric and pediatric units.

Nursing actions. The highest frequency categories of nursing actions for pediatric nurses in this sample were "adjusts I.V." (mean score 3.33), "T.P.R., blood pressure" (2.49), "straightens bedding, and so on" (2.38), and "touching, holding, cuddling, stroking" (2.24). Thus, pediatric nurses most frequently engaged in the routines of nursing care (for example, T.P.R.), various "straightening" behaviors, and maintained physical contact with their patients.

In general, pediatric nurses on the average, performed more nursing actions than did medical-surgical nurses. This was reflected, for example, in the fact that five categories of action occurred in more than 20 percent of the pediatric nurse-patient interactions, while no single category of action was as high as 20 percent for medical-surgical nurses.

The patterns of nursing actions for pediatric and obstetric nurses were similar in several respects, both groups showing high frequencies in adjusting patients' position, various "straightening" behaviors, and maintaining physical contact with their patients. There were, of course, obvious differences with respect to categories of action specific to obstetric nursing (for example, palpates abdomen, times contractions). In addition, obstetric nurses somewhat more often engaged in teaching and demonstrating actions (about 10 percent for obstetric nurses and less than 4 percent for pediatric nurses).

Differences between High and Low Inference Groups

Verbal interactions. Comparisons of verbal interactions for pediatric nurses in the high and low inference groups showed that of the categories relevant to expected differences, two revealed statistically significant differences: nurses in the high inference group chatted with their patients about their conditions and expressed sympathetic understanding and reassurance more frequently (both significant $p \leq .05$). None of the other relevant categories and none of the nonrelevant categories showed significant differences between the two groups.

Nursing actions. Statistically significant differences were obtained for three relevant categories: high inference nurses more frequently changed their patients' positions and provided physical nurturing, while low inference nurses more frequently engaged in "straightening" behavior (all significant $p \leq .05$). None of the other relevant and none of the nonrelevant categories revealed significant differences.

Relation to patient. Only one dimension of the comparisons of relation to patient for pediatric nurses showed a statistically significant difference: nurses in the high inference group were rated as somewhat warmer in emotional tone than were nurses in the low inference group (significant $p \leq .05$). None of the other dimensions revealed significant differences.

Discussion

Results for pediatric nurses showed a number of differences in the expected direction. Pediatric nurses who tended to infer relatively high patient suffering also tended to chat with their patients and express sympathetic understanding and reassurance more often; they appear to be more concerned with the comfort of their patients' positions, engaged more frequently in physical nurturing, and less often displayed "straightening" behavior. Finally, they were rated as emotionally warmer in their overall interactions with patients. Thus, data obtained for the sample of pediatric nurses clearly supported the proposition that nurses' beliefs about suffering were consistently and meaningfully related to their nursing behaviors.

Conclusions

To provide an overview of findings obtained in all three studies reported in this section, the statistically significant differences between nurses in the high and low inference groups are summarized in Table 13-1. An entry of *Yes* indicates that for a given category and a given setting, a significant difference was obtained in the comparison of high and low inference groups. An entry of *No* indicates that the difference found for the sample studied was not statistically significant. It should be noted that all of the significant differences found in the three studies and summarized in Table 13-1 were in the expected direction. Thus, for example, among medical-surgical nurses it was found that the high inference group more frequently defended and explained their actions to patients than did the low inference group; however, for this

Table 13-1
Summary of Statistically Significant Differences in
Expected Direction for Medical-Surgical,
Obstetric, and Pediatric Nurses

Category	Expected Difference	Medical-Surgical	Obstetric	Pediatric
Verbal Interactions				
Defends, explains actions	high > low	Yes	No	No
Dismisses patient's concerns	low > high	Yes	No	No
Verbalizes, explains actions to be taken	high > low	Yes	No	No
Sympathetic understanding, reassurance	high > low	No	Yes	Yes
Touching, holding, cuddling, stroking	high > low	*	Yes	No
Chats about condition	high > low	No	No	Yes
Nursing Actions				
Changes patient's position	high > low	Yes	No	Yes
Physical nurturing	high > low	No	Yes	No
Straightens bedding, and so on.	low > high	Yes	No	Yes
Relation to Patient				
Physical distance	high > low	Yes	No	No
Emotional tone	high > low	Yes	No	Yes
Amount of touching	high > low	Yes	No	No

*Not included in observational categories for this study.

category of verbal interaction, the differences found for both the obstetric sample and the pediatric sample were not significant.

Beliefs and behaviors. Inspection of Table 13-1 strongly suggests that there is indeed a relationship between nurses' beliefs about suffering and their nursing behavior. This is supported both by the number of positive findings and the fact that all of the significant differences obtained in the three studies are in the expected direction. Moreover, none of the categories that are not relevant to our initial expectations revealed statistically significant differences.

These findings add considerable weight to the results of previous investigations of nurses' reactions to suffering. In earlier studies we were primarily concerned with explicating nurses' implicit beliefs about suffering and determining those variables which influence reactions to the degree of pain and psychological distress experienced by patients. In the course of these investigations a substantial number of findings were obtained and a good deal was learned about nurses' beliefs about suffering. However, until the present research, the concept of nurses' implicit beliefs about suffering was not empirically tied to actual nursing behavior. It seemed reasonable, of course, to assume that nurses' beliefs were related to their behavior, but without clearcut empirical evidence, this assumption remained untested. Thus, the results of this investigation were not only interesting and valuable in terms of the specific issue studied, but they also validated the usefulness of our earlier research. By virtue of the present findings, the concept of nurses' implicit beliefs about suffering moved from an interesting theoretical construct to a variable that was directly and empirically tied to actual nursing practice. Prior to present research it was abundantly clear that this line of investigation was richly productive from a theoretical point of view. This productivity was demonstrated by the cumulative series of findings that clarified nurses' belief systems about suffering. These findings took on much greater significance when we knew that at least one major dimension of nurses' beliefs about suffering was consistently and meaningfully related to nursing behavior in interactions with patients.

Situational Differences

Although, in general, nurses' beliefs and behaviors are related, inspection of Table 13-1 suggests that the specific nature of the relationship depends upon the particular setting considered. In the three studies reported in this series, there were no single categories of either verbal interaction or nursing action and no single dimensions of relation to patient that revealed significant differences for nurses in all three settings. Medical-surgical nurses who tended to infer relatively high suffering in patients also tended to more frequently explain their actions to patients and to less frequently dismiss their patient's concerns. But among obstetric nurses, both high and low inference groups frequently explained their actions to patients and rarely dismissed the patients' concerns. Similarly, pediatric nurses who tended to infer relatively high suffering also tended more frequently to express sympathetic understanding and to chat about the patients' condition. But among medical-surgical nurses, neither high nor low inference nurses devoted much time to chatting with patients about their conditions and did not very frequently express sympathetic understanding and reassurance. Thus, the setting in which nurses worked had a very important impact on the ways in which their beliefs were reflected in their behaviors.

Support for this proposition was derived from a comparison of results for obstetric and medical-surgical nurses. In the medical-surgical setting, significant differences were obtained for three categories of verbal interactions, two categories of nursing actions, and three dimensions concerning nurse's relation to patient. In the obstetric setting, however, significant differences were obtained for only two categories of verbal interactions, one category of nursing actions, and for none of the dimensions dealing with relation to patient. For the medical-surgical nurse there was apparently a good deal of opportunity for beliefs to be expressed in behavior. There was often enough leeway in the medical-surgical unit to permit a range of adequate nursing behavior. For the obstetric nurse, however, the immediate demands of the working situation were likely to be much more restrictive on behavior. One could not remain physically distant from the patients; an inquiry about the patient's feelings had to have been made in order to perform appropriately; when the patient experienced pain, the evidence of this pain was obvious, and the nurse could not readily or reasonably dismiss the patient's concerns. Furthermore, the obstetric nurse's actions were likely to be determined largely by the patient's physical condition. In comparison to the medical-surgical nurse, the obstetric nurse had a relatively restricted range of tasks to perform. Situational factors probably exerted a greater influence on the obstetric nurse's behavior, and as a result, the relation between beliefs and behavior was more tenuous than that found for medical-surgical nurses.

Further evidence in support of the differential effects of various situations was derived from a consideration of the overall behavior of the combined groups of nurses in each of the three settings. Consider, for example, the pediatric versus the medical-surgical nurses. By and large, the pediatric nurses talked much more with the children who were their patients. They spent a good deal of time chatting with the children about their condition, exploring the children's feelings, and offering sympathetic understanding and reassurance. In contrast, the medical-surgical nurse much less often engaged in these kinds of verbal interactions. There was no evidence to support the assumption that medical-surgical nurses in comparison to pediatric nurses, were any less sensitive to or concerned about their patients, and there was no significant difference in their beliefs about suffering. It seemed most reasonable, therefore, to interpret the observed differences in nursing behaviors as a function of differences in the situations in which pediatric and medical-surgical nurses worked. Informal observations during the course of this research suggested that pediatric nurses had greater opportunity to talk with their patients, and informal chatting with the children in their unit was more likely to be viewed as an intrinsic part of pediatric nursing care. Medical-surgical nurses, on the other hand, appeared to have less opportunity for informal conversation with patients and seemed less likely to view such conversation as a significant part of their nursing responsibilities.

Theoretical Implications

From a theoretical point of view, the results of this series of studies tend to support an interpretation of low inferences of suffering as a reflection, in part, of a defensive or protective mechanism used by the nurse. This mechanism is similar to Harry Stack Sullivan's concept of "selective inattention" as a means of dealing with anxiety. According to Sullivan (1953), a commonly used technique for reducing anxiety is to pay selective inattention to the source of the threat. In colloquial terms, if you don't pay attention to the threat you won't feel so anxious—and maybe it will go away.

For some nurses, patients' suffering may be a source of threat that elicits anxiety. Forced to deal on a day-to-day basis with people who are in pain and experiencing psychological distress, and confronted by the fact that on some occasions the nurse cannot significantly relieve the patient's suffering, selective inattention to this suffering may be a very effective way for the nurse to maintain her own psychological integrity. Believing that patients do not suffer a great deal of pain or psychological distress is a form of selective inattention, and our measure of low inferences of suffering may reflect, in part, this mechanism. Just as the low inference nurse's belief system reflects this mechanism, so too does his or her nursing behavior reflect a tendency to pay selective inattention to the experiences of the patient. Thus, the low inference nurse may appear to act insensitively, though this behavior may be, in fact, a consequence of *sensitivity* to another person's suffering, and the anxiety that this suffering elicits in the nurse.

To a certain extent, most people who work closely with those who are suffering probably use one form or another of selective inattention. It is a common psychological mechanism in everyday life used to deal with anxiety-inducing situations, and there is no reason to believe that nurses are exempt from using this mechanism. A problem in nursing care arises, however, when this mechanism takes an extreme form. As indicated by this research, low inferences of suffering are associated with nursing behaviors that maintain psychological distance between nurse and patient. The psychologically distant nurse is less likely to take the patient's feelings into account and thus is probably less effective in relieving the patient's distress.

The problem for nursing, then, is to devise a means of guarding against overreactions to patient suffering that lead to psychologically protective mechanisms that, in turn, interfere with effective nursing care. This research offers no empirical basis for developing such safeguards, but the results of these investigations suggest that this is an important avenue for future research.

Methodological Implications

Although the substantive findings of this research are especially important, the methodological implications are also noteworthy. In research concerned with nursing, there has not been a great deal of investigation that has dealt directly with observations of actual nursing care. This is not to say that such research is entirely absent from nursing research literature, but by and large, relatively few investigators have reported studies in which the data have been obtained from observations of ongoing nurse-patient interactions. Therefore, in carrying out this study, the development of an appropriate method for obtaining observational data was necessarily based on a rather limited range of previous research. In this light, then, the present study makes a methodological, as well as substantive, contribution to nursing research. That is, the particular observational methods used in this study represent a potentially useful addition to the growing body of techniques concerned with direct observation of nursing behaviors. As nursing research continues to grow and expand, it seems likely that there will be an increasing need for such techniques. While the methods used in this study are unquesitonably limited in scope, the fact that they reveal meaningful relationships between beliefs and behavior lends credence to their potential value in future research.

Summary

In summary, this study successfully identifies certain relationships between nurses' general tendencies to infer either very high or very low suffering and specific nursing behavior. These findings are theoretically meaningful, and are especially important in that they link previous studies of nurses' belief systems to actual nursing practice. Moreover, this investigation provides a methodological contribution to a broader area of nursing research concerned with direct observation of nursing care. Nevertheless, care must be taken in generalizing the present results, recognizing that, while this study represents a significant step in the direction of enhancing our understanding of nursing behavior, useful generalizations in this area necessarily depend upon future research dealing with other aspects of nurses' beliefs about suffering and nursing behavior in other settings.

Part Six

Summary and Discussion

In this section a summary of findings is presented and the results discussed in relation to nursing practice, education, theory and research.

14
Summary of Findings

In the course of this research, a substantial number of empirical findings have been obtained. Before considering the theoretical and applied implications of the research, it would be useful to review and summarize the specific results of the various studies.

• Nurses' inferences of physical pain are consistently related to socioeconomic status of the patient, with lower status patients generally believed to suffer more pain than do patients of middle and upper socioeconomic status.

• Nurses' inferences of psychological distress are not consistently related to socioeconomic status of the patient. However, differences in amount of psychological distress associated with gender of the patient, nature of the illness, and degree of severity are indeed a function of the patient's socioeconomic status. Thus, while the socioeconomic variable in and of itself is a major determinant of nurses' inferences of physical pain, its effect on judgments of psychological distress is conditional by patient gender.

• In view of the consistently significant interaction effects obtained for both physical pain and psychological distress, it is apparent that nurses' belief systems regarding patient suffering involve a complex matrix of variables. For example, while a patient's socioeconomic status influences nurses' judgments about physical pain likely to be experienced by the patient, these judgments of pain are also conditioned by variables such as the patient's gender and the nature of the illness. Thus, in understanding a nurse's matrix of beliefs about physical pain, socioeconomic status of the patient must be considered in conjunction with the patient's gender and illness. Similarly a patient's socioeconomic status in interaction with other patient and illness

161

variables influences psychological distress. In general, then, it seems reasonable to conclude that the socioeconomic status of the patient is an important variable in nurses' belief systems about suffering, but represents only one part of a multi-dimensional matrix that must be taken into account in understanding inferences of both pain and psychological distress.

• The nature of the patient's illness in interaction with the patient's socioeconomic status accounts for a large part of the variance in nurses' reactions to suffering. This is true for both physical pain and psychological distress. Illustrating this proposition are the results obtained for cardiovascular illnesses. In their inferences of physical pain, nurses generally tend to see lower status patients as suffering more. But the reverse is true for cardiovascular illnesses. Nurses believe upper status cardiovascular patients suffer the most pain and lower status patients suffer the least pain. The same relationship between cardiovascular illness and socioeconomic status also appears to hold for inferences of psychological distress, in that upper status cardiovascular patients, in comparison to lower status patients, are viewed as suffering more psychological distress. The interaction between a patient's socioeconomic status and the nature of the patient's illness, therefore, plays a particularly important role in influencing nurses' inferences of suffering.

• Gender of the patient interacts with socioeconomic status in influencing nurses' reactions to suffering. For example, in their inferences of physical pain, nurses view lower status females as suffering more than lower status males, while for upper status patients the opposite is true. Once again, the complexity of nurses' belief systems about suffering is underscored by these interaction effects involving the patient's gender and socioeconomic status.

• Socioeconomic background of the nurse is not consistently related to reactions to suffering. However, this conclusion is tempered by the relatively restricted distribution of socioeconomic backgrounds among nurses in the sample studied. By and large, the majority of nurses in the sample come from middle and lower-middle class backgrounds. There are relatively few nurses at either end of the distribution. Therefore, comparisons of nurses on the basis of their own socioeconomic backgrounds involve subjects who were quite similar to one another along this dimension, and the null results obtained for this variable might well be accounted for by this restricted distribution.

• Age of the patient appears to have little influence on nurses' inferences of physical pain. However, age does play an important role in nurses' inferences of psychological distress.

• Nurses, in general, believe that children, ages 4–12, experience considerably less psychological distress than do patients in any older age group.

• Although children in general are seen as less distressed psychologically than patients in any other age group, nurses' perceptions of other age groups are influenced by the nature of the illness. Thus, the psychological distress experienced by the 17–25 and 65 + groups with psychiatric illnesses is seen as especially high, while 30–45-year-old patients are believed to experience particularly high distress in cases of cardiovascular disease.

• In studying the interaction of age with both severity and gender, the findings are that nurses tend to see children and the elderly in similar ways in comparison to the 17–25 and 30–45-year-old groups.

• As in the study of socioeconomic status, a large part of the variance in ratings of psychological distress is accounted for by the nature and severity of the illness. Each illness category shows a specific pattern of distress for the three levels of severity. For example, with the cancer category, there is little distress associated with the mild degree of illness, but nearly as much distress for the moderate level as there is for the severe level. In contrast, the amount of psychological distress inferred for a mild cardiovascular disease is relatively high, while the distress associated with infectious disease is not seen as very great until the illness is severe.

• Ethnic background of the patient is an important determinant of nurses' reactions to suffering. This is true for both physical pain and psychological distress.

• In general, for both dimensions of suffering, nurses see Jewish and Spanish patients as suffering most, and Oriental and Anglo-Saxon/Germanic patients as suffering least.

• The most consistent and striking difference among ethnic groups involves nurses' perceptions of Jewish patients as suffering relatively greater pain and psychological distress in cases of psychiatric and cardiovascular illnesses.

• In general, nurses tend to infer a greater degree of psychological distress than physical pain in evaluating the suffering typically associated with most illnesses and injuries.

• Over a wide variety of illnesses and injuries, nurses' inferences of psychological distress are independent of their inferences of physical pain. For some specific conditions, however, nurses do see a high congruence between physical pain and psychological distress. This seems to be particularly true for severe trauma and severe cardiovascular illnesses; in these cases, a high degree of suffering is inferred along both dimensions. For other mild or clearly treatable conditions, little physical or psychological suffering is inferred.

• Conditions viewed as physically most painful tend to involve severe trauma or cardiovascular illnesses, though specific conditions outside of these two broad categories are also seen as particularly painful.

• In addition to various psychiatric illnesses, physical illnesses or injuries seen as psychologically most distressful typically involve the threat of death or long-term, severe disability.

• The tendency of a nurse, in comparison to other nurses, to infer relatively high or low suffering in patients is a stable characteristic that can be measured reliably by the *Standard Measure of Inference of Suffering* developed in the course of this project. Thus, in considering various kinds of patients and a variety of illnesses and injuries, some nurses consistently infer a relatively high degree of suffering and some nurses consistently infer relatively lower degrees of suffering.

• The race of the nurse does not influence the degree of physical pain inferred, and there is no interaction between the race of the nurse and the race of the patient in reactions to pain.

•Black nurses tend to infer a greater degree of psychological distress than do White nurses; however, the race of the patient does not appear to influence the nurses differentially.

• Nurses from various countries (United States, Japan, Puerto Rico, Korea, Thailand, Taiwan) differ in their inferences of both physical pain and psychological suffering. In comparison to nurses in other countries, American nurses tend to infer relatively low physical pain and moderate psychological distress.

• There is a significant interaction between nature of the illness or injury and national background in nurses' reactions to suffering. For example, Korean nurses infer the greatest pain for traumatic injuries, while Japanese nurses infer the greatest pain for cancer.

• There is a significant interaction between age of the patient and national background in nurses' inferences of suffering. For example, Japanese nurses infer the greatest pain for children, while American nurses infer the greatest pain for elderly patients.

• In general, nurses in all of the countries studied tend to see female patients, in comparison with male patients, as suffering somewhat more physical pain and psychological distress. There is a significant interaction between sex and national background for inferences of physical pain; however, this interaction is not significant for psychological distress.

• In their retrospective reports, nurses describe a change in their reactions to patients during the course of their training and practice. They often explain this change as a shift from the idealism of school to the realism of practice, a shift from a sense of universal sympathy to more controlled and selective reactions to specific patients.

• While nurses described themselves as becoming more realistic and discriminating in their reactions to patients' suffering, they also described themselves as becoming more compassionate and understanding. Thus, in contrast to their more general sympathetic reactions at the beginning of training, experienced nurses report a more selective, but also more sensitive response to particular patients.

• Nurses in general are aware of their special sensitivities to particular kinds of patients. For some nurses, age of the patient is a crucial factor determining their response. Nature of the illness appears to be an important determinant for almost all nurses, with the most intense sympathetic response elicited by patients who are severely disabled or likely to die.

• Most nurses report a clear distinction between those patients "who have a right to complain" and those who are merely "complainers." Thus, if a patient says that he is suffering, but a nurse infers relatively little pain or psychological distress, the patient is often labeled "a complainer." These patients tend to elicit irritation, anger, and rejection on the part of the nurse, and these emotional reactions are sometimes accompanied by guilt.

• In general, nurses tend to report the greatest difficulty in dealing with patients who have emotional problems. Part of this difficulty appears to be a consequence of the nurse's sense of inadequacy in alleviating psychological distress.

• Many nurses are concerned about being overwhelmed by the suffering of patients with whom they have close contact. This is associated with the problem of a nurse's over-involvement with a particular patient, and many nurses describe traumatic experiences involving patients with whom they become over-involved early in their professional careers. As a result of these early experiences, most nurses develop various ways of establishing some emotional distance between themselves and their patients.

• Of all the problems encountered by the nurses, the death of a patient is emotionally the most devastating for the majority of nurses. One of the most common reactions reported by nurses is a desire to escape from the situation, minimizing contact with a dying patient.

• Nurses who tend to infer relatively high physical pain also tend to infer relatively high psychological distress.

• Nurses who tend to infer relatively high pain in patients also tend to report personal experiences that are relatively painful. Thus, reported sensitivity to pain in one's own life is associated with the inference of greater pain experienced by others.

• Nurses who tend to infer relatively high physical pain tend to augment various kinds of stimulation.

• Nurses who tend to infer relatively high psychological distress tend to prefer interpersonal rather than more technical nursing activities.

• The degree of suffering inferred by nurses, including inferences of both pain and psychological distress, is independent of the tendency to repress one's own feelings of anxiety, reported stoic attitudes, years of professional experience, current nursing position, or area of nursing specialization. However, nurses who tend to infer relatively little suffering come from North European family backgrounds more often than would be expected by chance. In contrast, nurses who tend to infer relatively high suffering tend to come from either South European or African family backgrounds more often than would be expected by chance.

• Nurses' beliefs about suffering are related to their nursing behavior in interactions with patients. In general, nurses who infer relatively high degrees of suffering among their patients, in comparison to those who infer less suffering, exhibit behavior that reflects greater concern with interpersonal and comforting aspects of nursing care. On the other hand, nurses who infer relatively low degrees of suffering tend to exhibit behavior that is less supportive of patients' complaints and is physically and emotionally more distant.

• Although, in general, nurses' beliefs and behavior are related, the specific nature of the relationship depends upon the particular setting considered. By and large, the relation between beliefs about suffering and nursing behavior is more clearly evident among medical-surgical and pediatric nurses than among obstetric nurses. It would seem that the situational demands of obstetric nursing are somewhat more compelling than those in medical-surgical or pediatric nursing, and thus, the relation between beliefs and behavior may be obscured in the obstetric setting.

• Students' beliefs about suffering change over the course of nursing education. In general, after their first year of training they tend to infer higher psychological distress and lower physical pain than they did upon entering nursing. These changes appear to occur during the first year of nursing education, and after the first year the level of inferences for both pain and psychological distress remains stable.

15

Implications of Findings

Various implications of this research have been suggested in the discussion of
each of the specific studies carried out in the course of this research. In this
final chapter, however, it may be useful to review briefly some of the more
general implications derived from the findings. These will be considered in
terms of nursing practice, the education of nurses, and nursing theory and
research.

Implications for Nursing Practice

Shared Beliefs

The initial studies in the project focused on the commonalities of belief
shared by the nurses sampled, and indeed, a number of these commonalities
were discovered. The fact that nurses more or less share beliefs about suffering raises important questions about the development of belief systems
within the profession. To a certain extent, the beliefs of American nurses
probably reflect the beliefs of the larger American culture. For example, the
belief that Oriental patients suffer less than others do is congruent with the
more general view of Orientals as stoic and relatively insensitive to pain—a
stereotype, incidentally, that is in marked contrast to our findings for nurses
in several Asian countries. In addition to the broader cultural influence,
however, the beliefs shared by nurses probably reflect common experiences
in training and practice, and may be viewed as part of the "culture" of professional nursing. Nurses' beliefs about the nature and degree of suffering
associated with various illnesses and injuries is an important case in point.
The patient's condition is a most important determinant of nurses' reactions
to suffering, and while this may partly reflect broader cultural beliefs about
various illnesses and injuries, nurses' professional experiences in caring for

patients who are ill or injured undoubtedly provide a major basis for the development of their beliefs about suffering. From this point of view, then, nurses' implicit belief systems are based on the realities of their day to day professional experiences. They have worked with patients who have cardiovascular illnesses or infectious diseases, and in the process of caring for these patients, nurses develop certain beliefs that are more or less shared within the profession. It is important, therefore, to recognize the reality or experiential basis of nurses' common beliefs about suffering.

One must also appreciate the value of these beliefs in nursing practice. If a nurse has learned, on the basis of previous experience, that a particular illness is associated with a great deal of pain or psychological distress, it is likely that the nurse will be sensitized to the suffering of a patient with this illness. This kind of sensitivity may indeed be a most important component of effective nursing care.

Just as nurses' implicit belief systems may sensitize them to the suffering associated with certain illnesses, it may also desensitize them to the suffering that may be associated with other illnesses. For example, nurses generally view epilepsy with grand mal seizures as an illness characterized by only moderate psychological distress, a belief presumably based, at least in part, on their experiences with epileptic patients. In dealing with these patients, therefore, nurses would probably not be especially concerned with or sensitive to the psychological distress that may be involved with this illness. In many cases, this lack of special concern may be quite appropriate and congruent with patients' feelings. However, there are epileptic patients who suffer intense psychological distress, and nurses' beliefs that this illness does not typically involve a high degree of psychological suffering may desensitize them to the feelings of particular patients.

The nurses we studied came from many different backgrounds and had a wide range of professional training and experience; nevertheless, despite these personal and professional differences, their judgments about the suffering of patients with various illnesses and injuries showed a good deal of agreement.

In view of these findings, one might think of beliefs about suffering as part of the *professional subculture* of nursing. An important feature that partly defines any group that can be considered a distinct subculture is a shared set of beliefs, and the results of our research indicate that nurses do indeed share a more or less common set of beliefs concerning patients' suffering. To a large extent, this sharing of beliefs probably reflects common experiences that nurses have regardless of their differing backgrounds. One nurse might specialize in pediatric care, another in obstetrics, and a third in medical-surgical nursing. But in the course of their training and professional careers, they are likely to share enough common experiences to develop a shared set of beliefs about the suffering experienced by patients with various illnesses or injuries.

In addition, nurses also "teach" each other the beliefs they come to share. By "teaching" we don't mean a formal kind of instruction that we usually associate with school, but rather, the kind of informal teaching and learning that occurs every day when we share our experiences with one another. For example, a nurse cares for a patient who has pre-infarction angina, and in conversations with other nurses talks about the pain as well as psychological distress the patient is experiencing. In this sense, then, he or she is "teaching" others on the basis of his or her own experiences, and as a result of mutual teaching of this sort, nurses develop a shared set of beliefs.

This kind of informal teaching is an important and often valuable part of every nurse's professional education. As a consequence of sharing experiences, nurses broaden the range of one another's professional competencies. Even though a nurse may not previously have cared for a patient with a pre-infarction angina, by virtue of sharing of experiences with other nurses, he or she will have some expectations about the pain and psychological distress such a patient is likely to suffer. This is clearly an advantage derived from the nurse's participation in the subculture of nursing.

Recognizing the potential advantages of the shared beliefs that are part of the nursing subculture, it is also important to appreciate the fact that patients do not necessarily share this subculture. From the patient's perspective, the degree of pain or psychological distress he or she is experiencing may be quite different from the level of suffering nurses might assume to be associated with the patient's particular illness. In the system of beliefs that nurses share, a draining abscess of the foot is not associated with a very high level of psychological distress. Nevertheless, for a particular patient this condition may be exceedingly threatening and evoke a good deal of anxiety. Thus, nurses' beliefs can serve to sensitize a nurse to the suffering a patient is likely to experience, but special care must be taken to make sure that these beliefs do not interfere with the nurse's accurate perception of an individual patient. The beliefs shared by nurses are an important and potentially valuable part of their professional subculture, but in the final analysis, it is the nurse's understanding of each particular patient that is crucial in determining the quality of nursing care provided.

The Patient's Socioeconomic Status

The results of this research clearly indicate that a patient's socioeconomic status influences nurses' beliefs about the suffering likely to be experienced by that patient. Socioeconomic status is undoubtedly a pervasive variable that influences attitudes and expectations along a wide variety of dimensions. In this respect, therefore, nurses' beliefs in relation to socioeconomic status probably reflect a much wider set of beliefs shared by many in the larger American culture. For nursing, however, these beliefs can make an enormous difference in the care given to patients. If a nurse believes that a cleaning woman with a broken arm suffers more pain than a wealthy fashion designer with exactly the same injury, it is more than likely that the nurse will pay particular attention to the cleaning woman's pain and perhaps even discount the pain of the woman who is a fashion designer. Yet, both women are patients, each experiences some degree of pain, and each deserves the nurse's individual attention and professional care regardless of their differences in socioeconomic status.

Similarly, the bank president and the laborer with a myocardial infarction may both be experiencing psychological distress that has little or nothing to do with how much money they have, how big or small a house they live in, or what part of town they come from. Each may feel threatened by the illness in his or her own way, and each should receive the nursing care needed. If a nurse believes that wealthier people suffer more psychological distress than do poorer people, he or she may well emphasize psychological aspects of care with wealthier patients and perhaps neglect this aspect of nursing care with less well-to-do patients.

Thus, in their professional role, nurses cannot permit the beliefs, biases, and stereotypes that operate in everyday life to influence their nursing care. Every patient is an individual who experiences his or her own unique pain and unique psychological distress, and effective nursing must be based on a recognition of each patients' individuality.

The findings of our research, therefore, suggest that each nurse should examine his or her own beliefs about patients from different social statuses. As a result of this self-examination a nurse may become aware of his or her own particular beliefs and biases, and on the basis of this awareness, guard against stereotypes that sometimes interfere with providing the nursing care that is best for each individual patient.

The Patient's Age

The results of our study show that nurses, in general, believe that when children are ill or injured, they suffer less psychological distress than adults with equivalent illnesses or injuries. Our discussions with nurses suggest that this judgment is based on the assumption that children do not understand as fully as adults the consequences and possible implications of their physical condition.

This finding and the reasoning underlying nurses' judgments about children clearly reflect an adult's point of view. For an adult, the psychological distress associated with illness may be based largely on concerns about what will happen as a result of the illness. The person's life may be more or less seriously disrupted, there may be some long-term disability involved, financial worries may add to the stress, and in some conditions, the possibility of death may be a source of anxiety. All of this, of course, requires some degree of understanding. Thus, from an adult's perspective, one might reason that, if children understand less about the implications and possible consequences of their conditions, they are less likely to worry about what might happen. In this sense, then, children's lack of knowledge and understanding may protect them from psychological distress.

Although this reasoning undoubtedly has some validity, it neglects the very important possibility that the major source of a child's anxiety may be somewhat different from that of adults. Separation from parents and the unfamiliar environment of the hospital can be extremely threatening to a child and give rise to intense fear. The lack of understanding of what is happening, plus the pain, and for the child, the mysterious events sometimes encountered during hospitalization can make the child extremely anxious.

In our observations and discussions with pediatric nurses, it is clear that the great majority of nurses who work primarily with children are well aware of these possible sources of psychological distress among children. On the basis of their experiences, they recognize that ill or injured children can very well be anxious as any adult patient, and effective pediatric care depends, in part, on sensitivity to this distress. Our study, however, indicates that other nurses, those who work largely with adults, may not empathize as fully as they might with children. As a result, there may be some tendency to discount the degree of psychological distress experienced by young patients. It would therefore be important to recognize that the causes of fear, anxiety, and worry for adults and children may sometimes differ, but both children and adults may suffer equivalent degrees of psychological distress regardless of differences in age.

The Patient's Ethnic and Cultural Background

The results of this study clearly show that the ethnic or cultural background of the patient influences the nurses' judgments about suffering. Six patients, each from a different ethnic background, with identical illnesses or injuries, were judged differently. The one factor, ethnic background, made a significant difference in the ratings.

We may reasonably ask, to what extent do preconceived attitudes about a specific ethnic group affect our behavior? Appreciating the particular characteristics of a given ethnic group certainly may be helpful. For example, one nurse stated, "Knowing Puerto Rican patients react a lot helps me. I expect them to make their complaints known. I try to stay one step ahead of them. I never have any problems because I am there first."

On the other hand, there may be times when the judgments 'get in the way' of relationships, particularly in those situations where the patient does not conform to the stereotypes. The Jewish man we spoke to had the feeling that the nurses expected him to complain. He felt they reacted to him as if he were demanding. In this instance, the nurses' belief system interfered with the development of a helpful nurse-patient relationship.

The problem for nursing is not simply a matter of doing away with all of our stereotypes. On the basis of previous research (for example, Zborowski, 1969), we know that patients from various ethnic groups tend to react differently to the kinds of stress encountered when they are ill or injured. By and large Oriental patients, for example, generally tend to react more stoically than do Puerto Rican patients. In itself, this difference is neither good nor bad; it is a reflection of the kinds of behavior expected of people in the two cultures. In general, a more stoic attitude towards pain is viewed as desirable in many Oriental cultures, while in the Puerto Rican culture a person is expected to be more emotionally expressive.

Being aware of these cultural differences can be helpful to the nurse because he or she can learn to understand the behavior of his or her patients in terms of their particular background. Thus, the nurse who is aware of cultural differences and understands the patients in terms of their cultural backgrounds will respond more appropriately and effectively to the patients' needs. The nurse will not be disturbed by the emotional expressiveness of a patient whose culture expects and encourages people to be very expressive, nor will he or she mistake a more stoic attitude among patients from a different culture for a lack of feelings.

Nevertheless, any generalization about a cultural or ethnic group of people can blind us to differences among individuals within that group. It may be true that Chinese patients as a group are more stoic than Puerto Rican patients as a group. But within any group there are enormous individual differences that must be recognized and appreciated by the nurse. In providing effective nursing care, the pain, psychological distress, and the needs of the *individual* patient must be taken into account. Thus, even though there may be certain similarities among members of a particular ethnic group, the nurse must be especially careful not to permit a stereotyped belief to interfere with sensitivity for the individual patient.

Our research findings indicate that nurses do share more or less common beliefs about the suffering experienced by patients from different ethnic, national, and religious backgrounds. These beliefs may be based on common experiences with patients from these various groups or they may stem from stereotypes people share in the larger American culture. But regardless of the basis of these beliefs, in providing health care nurses must be sensitive to the individuals who are their patients. Therefore, an important step in gaining this sensitivity to individuals is becoming aware of one's own generalized beliefs. If a nurse is aware of his or her own beliefs about groups of people, he or she can then guard against these generalizations distorting any judgments about *individuals.* Through this kind of self-awareness and self-knowledge nurses can achieve the awareness and understanding of others that is crucial in providing effective nursing care.

The Nurse's Cultural Background

While the initial studies in this project dealt primarily with the common beliefs about suffering shared by American nurses, the later phases of the research focused on individual and group differences among nurses. In this respect, our research indicated that cultural or national backgrounds played a significant part in determining nurses' reactions to suffering. American nurses clearly differed from nurses in other countries, and even within the American groups, ethnic and national background of a nurse affect the inferences made about patients. Thus, for example, black American nurses and those whose family backgrounds were South European tended to infer more suffering than did nurses whose family backgrounds were North European. From these data it was evident that beliefs about suffering were, in part, socially learned, and the particular cultural context in which that learning occured made a significant difference in a nurse's reactions to patients' experiences.

The implications of these findings are especially important in settings which involve the interaction of nurses and patients from different cultural and national backgrounds. The congruence of a nurse's inference about a patient's suffering and the patient's own interpretation and evaluation of his or her experience depends, in part, on the degree to which they share common views about pain and psychological distress. If a nurse comes from a cultural background that prizes stoicism and discounts the intensity of suffering associated with illness or injury, that nurse is not likely to respond with a great deal of empathic understanding to patients whose cultural background differs markedly in this respect. Thus, the nurse with an Anglo-Saxon/Germanic background may have some difficulty empathizing with the patient whose background is Mediterranean.

At the present time, this is an issue of considerable significance in nursing practice, particularly in American metropolitan hospitals. Both nurses and patients in these hospitals come from a wide variety of cultural backgrounds, and as a consequence there may be some difficulty in communication among nurses as well as between nurses and their patients. This is not primarily a difficulty stemming from linguistic differences, but rather, from differences in beliefs about the nature and intensity of suffering associated with illness and injury.

Simply noting these differences does not, in and of itself, automatically resolve the differences and lead to empathic understanding. However, recognizing that inferences of another person's experience are based on beliefs about pain and psychological distress, and that these beliefs are culture-bound is an important first step in moving towards a greater congruence between nurses' inferences and patients' experiences. If nurses realize that their own beliefs are culture-bound, they may become increasingly aware of possible differences between their own inferences and patients' experiences, and on the basis of this awareness, adjust or "recalibrate" their judgments about patients to take into account culturally derived interpretations of the nature and intensity of suffering. As a result, nurses may become more sensitive to their patients' feelings, more accurate in their evaluations of patients' experiences of pain and psychological distress, and more effective in dealing with patients' suffering.

Helping the Nurse Gain Greater Self-Awareness— A Practical Step

As our research has indicated, part of the "professional subculture" of American nursing involves more or less shared beliefs about the nature and degree of suffering associated with various illnesses, injuries, and patient characteristics. We have not argued that these beliefs, in general, are either "right" or "wrong"; in fact, we have no evidence about the validity of any of the beliefs about suffering that are commonly held by the nurses we studied. Nevertheless, any stereotyped belief about the experiences of others is bound to obscure individual differences among people.

The most effective countermeasure for dealing with stereotyped beliefs is self-knowledge. This implies the need for systematic self-examination by nurses of their own implicit belief systems. Such self-examination is not easy to pursue, and superficial self-study is not likely to produce results that are practically worthwhile. Therefore, to achieve this kind of self-awareness, it would seem desirable to introduce institutional means of buttressing nurses' independent efforts to gain self-awareness.

For example, it might be useful for a given hospital to organize short-term self-study groups among nurses on the staff to examine their own beliefs, share opinions and experiences, identify their own stereotypes, and in the process of interacting with other nurses, modify and change these stereotypes and become more aware of individual differences among patients.

Bringing these implicit beliefs to the level of conscious awareness and making them explicit for oneself and for others is an important first step in achieving perception of patients' feelings. These kinds of self-study groups are not, of course, a panacea, and it must be recognized that groups of nurses who share the same belief system may reinforce each other's stereotypes. Nevertheless, some systematic means of self-study would undoubtedly be of considerable value as part of a nurse's program of continuing professional education.

The Psychological Distance between Nurse and Patient

The practical significance of this line of investigation is considerably enhanced by the research demonstrating a consistent and meaningful relationship between reactions to suffering and nursing behavior in interactions with patients. The specific findings have been discussed in conjunction with our report of that particular study. At this point, only the more general implications of these findings need be considered.

Nurses who infer relatively low suffering in their patients, in comparison to those who infer relatively high suffering, tend to be emotionally and physically more distant from their patients. We have interpreted this emotional and physical distance as a reflection of a psychological defense mechanism aimed at protecting the nurse from the stress induced by daily, close contact with the suffering of others. From this point of view, inferences of relatively low suffering are not the consequence of insensitivity or callousness. Rather, they reflect a defensive reaction to the potential threat of too great a sensitivity to the suffering of others.

One might recall our interviews with nurses who described the trauma of becoming overly involved with their patients. In these instances, the psychological distance between nurse and patient was reduced, and as a consequence, the nurses empathically shared their patients' pain and psychological distress. Many of these nurses said, "never again," and in one way or another developed mechanisms for establishing psychological distance between themselves and their patients. Without these mechanisms, the nurses' own psychological stability would be threatened and their professional effectiveness inevitably reduced.

One of these mechanisms involves the belief that the patients with whom one works really are not suffering too badly. This permits the nurse to remain emotionally and physically distant from the patient, reduces the potential threat to the nurse, and allows the maintenance of a reasonable degree of professional integrity as well as personal stability. In terms of the nurse's own psychological functioning, minimizing the suffering of those with whom the nurse must come into close contact as an intrinsic part of daily professional life is an "emotionally reasonable" means of adapting to the stresses inherent in much of nursing.

If we are concerned only with the nurse's emotional integration, various means of maintaining psychological distance from patients may be evaluated primarily in terms of their effectiveness in reducing stress. However, the nurse's principal professional responsibility is the care of patients, and as our research has indicated, the nature of this care is influenced by the nurse's inferences about his or her patients. One cannot conclude that the nurses who were emotionally and physically more distant from the patient necessarily provided less effective nursing care. Nevertheless, it seems reasonable to assume that, in general, a nurse who behaves as if he or she were insensitive to patients' suffering is not likely to offer optimal nursing care. Perhaps too much empathy on the part of a nurse interferes with carrying out professional responsibilities. But at the other extreme, acting as if one were unaware of the pain and psychological distress experienced by patients is hardly conducive to providing the human quality of care that goes beyond technical proficiency.

We come, then, to a central issue in nursing. On the one hand, sensitivity to the feelings of patients is essential for effective nursing care. On the other hand, some psychological distance between nurse and patient is necessary for the nurse's own emotional adjustment and continuing professional effectiveness. By virtue of his or her professional role, the nurse faces something of a dilemma: one must be both emotionally sensitive to, as well as somewhat distant from the patients with whom one works. An effective nurse, therefore, must somehow resolve this dilemma, integrating both the need for sensitivity and the need to maintain some psychological distance.

Our research at this stage does not offer an empirical basis for resolving this issue. However, recognition of this central problem in nursing highlights the importance of studying the professional development of nurses in terms of their reactions to patients' pain and psychological distress. As we have suggested earlier, nurses' beliefs about suffering are a major part of the professional subculture of nursing, and it is within the framework of this subculture that a nurse must deal with the dilemma of maintaining both sensitivity to and distance from patients.

Implications for Nursing Education

Sensitivity to Psychological Distress

Nursing educators have focused a good deal of effort on the goal of sensitizing nursing students to the feelings of patients. These educational efforts are reflected, for example, in recent curriculum developments that emphasize a psychological understanding of the effects of illness and hospitalization and more explicit consideration of the interpersonal aspects of nursing. The results of our study of changes in beliefs over the course of nursing education clearly indicate that these efforts have been successful. Nursing students unquestionably become increasingly aware of their patients' psychological distress.

The general aim of these educational developments is certainly worthwhile, and the present research does not raise any question about the general goal of educating nurses to become aware of their patients' feelings. However, our research suggests that, in nursing practice, the nurse's sensitivity to patients' suffering must be considered in conjunction with the nurse's own emotional stability and adjustment to a potential stressful situation. For many nurses who practice in hospital settings, the suffering of others is a fact of daily life, and a good deal of their nursing practice is concerned directly with the pain and psychological distress of patients. Given this situation, a nurse who responded with great empathic sensitivity to all of the suffering encountered in daily practice would soon be psychologically in an impossible position. As we indicated earlier, for the sake of the nurse's own emotional and professional adjustment, sensitivity to the suffering of others must be tempered by some degree of psychological distance between the nurse and the patient.

Thus, nursing educators must recognize that sensitivity is a two-edged sword that can lead to more effective nursing practice, but may also result in emotional stress that seriously disrupts the nurse's personal and professional functioning. Focusing educational efforts only in the direction of increasing sensitivity to patients' feelings emphasizes only one aspect of the complex issue nurses face in practice, and in the long run, may result in less, rather than more, effective nursing.

This implies that nursing educators must help their students deal explicitly with the issue of integrating the need to be sensitive to patients' feelings and the need to maintain appropriate psychological distance from patients. There is probably no single, best way of resolving this issue, and at this stage of our research we cannot offer concrete guidelines for dealing with this problem. However, it may be important for nursing educators to recognize that a curriculum designed to increase nursing students' awareness of patient's psychological distress is not enough. Nursing education must also help students understand their defensive reactions to the suffering of others, including the defense of distancing themselves from patients, and on the basis of this knowledge, develop a professional stance that combines both emotional sensitivity to patients' feelings with appropriate psychological distance between nurse and patient. In addition, nursing students must also have an opportunity to acquire techniques for responding to patients' psychological distress that are not only effective, but also realistically practical in actual settings of nursing practice. This problem, which must be faced by nursing researchers as well as nursing educators, will be considered in greater detail in a subsequent section of this chapter dealing with nursing research.

Sensitivity to Pain

The results of our research indicate that over the course of their education, nursing students' reactions to patients' physical pain tend to decrease. This finding is in sharp contrast to the results for psychological distress and reflect the divergent patterns of change in beliefs about these two aspects of suffering.

We cannot, of course, evaluate the validity of these changes in beliefs, but considering the data at face value, it is apparent that there is a significant decrease in the level of patient pain inferred by students as they gain academic and clinical experience in nursing. To some extent, this change in beliefs reflects the students' increasing knowledge of medication and nursing procedures that effectively relieve patients' pain. They learn about these measures in their academic studies and clinical training and have an opportunity to observe their effectiveness. As a result, they appreciate the fact that pain can be relieved by appropriate nursing, and this knowledge is reflected in the reduced level of their inferences of pain.

Although the observed changes in nursing students' beliefs about pain are a valid result of what they have learned, these changes may eventually lead to a desensitization of the student which may interfere with subsequent nursing behavior. No matter how effective pain-relief measures might be, the effective nurse cannot view the pain experienced by an individual patient as a routine matter to be dealt with only by standardized, technical means. Thus, nursing educators must guard against potential over-desensitization among their students, achieving a balance between extreme sensitivity and under-sensitivity to patients' pain.

In this regard it may be useful for nursing educators to note our finding of the positive relationship between nurses' reactions to patients' pain and nurses' own experiences of pain. This finding has certain implications for the education of nurses. It certainly does *not* mean that nurses have to suffer themselves in order to empathize with the suffering of their patients. But it does suggest that in one way or another, a nurse should learn about the experience of pain. Personal experience with pain is only one way in which this can be achieved. We also learn from the experience of others if we pay attention to these experiences, listen to what others say, and read what others have written. For example, people who have suffered a great deal of pain, as a result of illness, injury or some other circumstances, have written about their experiences, and reading these reports can serve as a very effective way of learning about other people's feelings. Similarly, as part of a nurse's education it may be important to devote a certain amount of time to exploring patients' experiences, and finding out in detail how they are feeling. Probably most, if not all, nurses do this as part of their training, but it may be worthwhile to introduce this kind of exploration of patients' feelings as a regular, systematic part of training throughout a nurse's professional education.

Implications for Nursing Theory

The results of this research incontrovertibly demonstrate the usefulness of conceptualizing the implicit belief system underlying nurses' reactions to suffering in terms of a matrix of variables involving both observed and inferred dimensions. From our theoretical point of view, we assume that nurses have an implicit matrix of beliefs relevant to suffering, a matrix that may be thought of, metaphorically, in the same general format as the usual matrix of intercorrelations commonly found in statistical analyses. We do not mean, of course, that individuals in fact compute correlations as a basis for establishing their belief systems. Presumably, these belief systems develop as a consequence of the individual's experience, without the kind of systematic treatment implied by the term statistical analysis.[68]" Our concern at this point is with the matrix of beliefs that guides a nurse's inferences, regardless of how that matrix was developed, and perhaps our most general conclusion is that the general idea of a belief matrix is a very useful theoretical concept. Beginning with this basic construct, our research led to a substantial number of findings that clarified nurses' reactions to suffering, and finally resulted in establishing a relationship between these kinds of reactions and actual nursing behavior in interactions with patients. Thus, the concept of a belief matrix is useful both in terms of the development of research as well as in understanding nursing practice. In fact, on the basis of our experience in this project, it would not be unreasonable to suggest that the concept of an implicit belief matrix may very well be a particularly useful theoretical idea for integrating nursing research and practice.

Complexity of Belief Systems

Although the implicit belief of matrix model does seem to be useful in this area of research, the matrices underlying nurses' beliefs are undoubtedly more complex than initially anticipated. This complexity is suggested by the consistently significant interaction effects found in the data, indicating that one variable modulates the effects of a second variable on judgments of suffering. For example, the overall analysis for patient's socioeconomic status revealed that, in general, nurses tended to see lower status patients as suffering more physical pain than middle or upper status patients. However, further analysis of the interaction between illnesses and socioeconomic status showed that, for cardiovascular illnesses, the general trend was reversed: upper status cardiovascular patients were seen as experiencing the greatest pain. In this instance, the effect of socioeconomic status on reactions to suffering was modulated by the nature of the illness.

These findings indicate that a simple two-dimensional model composed of a series of discrete relationships between a particular observable variable and a particular inference is inadequate for the purposes of understanding nursing behavior. Rather, a multidimensional model that takes into account the variety of interactions found in our data is needed for an adequate conceptualization of the results.

A patient's age, sex, socioeconomic status, and illness or injury are clearly important variables that influence nurses' reactions to suffering. The specific findings regarding each of these variables have been discussed at some length in preceding sections of this chapter. At this point it is important to note that none of these variables operates independently of others. The effect of sex is modulated by the patient's socioeconomic status; the effect of illness or injury is a function of the patient's age. Therefore, while each of the major variables thus far considered contributes to the overall variance in nurses' reactions to suffering, it is most meaningful to interpret their effects in terms of complex interactions in which the influence of one variable is modulated by other variables.

Other Relevant Beliefs

The development of a general theory of nursing is obviously beyond the scope of this book. The results of our research, however, suggest that the concept of an implicit belief matrix should be an important component of any such theory.

In this project, we were concerned with implicit beliefs about suffering, and the results of the research provided ample evidence of the theoretical usefulness of this construct. In developing a general theory of nursing, however, this construct might well be expanded to include other kinds of beliefs relevant to nursing. For example, beliefs about the causes of illness and about the effectiveness of therapeutic measures might be important determinants of nursing behavior that could usefully be included in a theory of nursing.

As a part of their education, nurses of course learn about the causes of illness and basis of various therapeutic measures, but in the course of practice, they also develop certain implicit beliefs about illness and therapy that influence their behavior. Thus, a consideration of these implicit beliefs may prove to be significant in developing a meaningful theory of nursing.

A nurse's implicit belief system may be viewed in terms of the processing of information involved in nursing. That is, in caring for a patient, a nurse confronts an enormous variety of complex and potentially significant stimuli which she must selectively perceive and interpret. In part, one's selective perceptions and interpretations are based upon implicit beliefs about what is important in a given situation and the meanings of various cues. For example, a nurse may implicitly believe that the age of a patient is an important determinant of the patient's reaction to illness. Thus, in dealing with patients, one may pay particular attention to the patient's age and interpret the patients' behavior as a function of age. If one believes that children experience relatively little psychological distress, one may pay selective inattention to a child's expressions of psychological suffering and interpret the child's behavior primarily in terms of physical discomfort or as a sign of misbehavior. In any event, regardless of the nurse's particular interpretation or response, the nurse's beliefs about suffering provide a basis for processing the information derived from the nurse-patient interaction.

We are not by any means suggesting that the nurse's implicit belief system is the only basis for information processing. Obviously, the nurse's technical knowledge also determines the way in which he or she processes information. However, without discounting the importance of technical or scientific knowledge, our research clearly demonstrates that a nurse's implicit beliefs about suffering significantly influence the nature of interactions with patients. In developing a general theory of nursing, therefore, the concept of implicit belief systems that operate in processing information appears to have a good deal of theoretical value.

Relating Beliefs to Behaviors

Although this research demonstrates the importance of considering nurses' beliefs as part of a general theory of nursing, the findings of the three studies relating beliefs to behaviors underscore the significance of situational factors. On the basis of our investigations, it is clear that a nurse's beliefs influence interactions with patients. But it is equally evident that the manner in which beliefs are reflected in behavior is a function of the particular setting considered. In a general medical-surgical unit, in contrast to other hospital units, there are likely to be relatively fewer constraints on acceptable nursing behavior, and one typically observes a wider range of behavior among nurses on such a unit. In this sense, therefore, there is a greater opportunity for a particular nurse's beliefs to be manifested in his or her behaviors. In an obstetric unit, however, the situation itself places more restrictive demands on a nurse's behavior, and thus allows somewhat less opportunity to observe the relation between beliefs and behaviors. In this situation, nursing actions are largely determined by physical cues indicative, for example, of the progress of labor, rather than by a nurse's interpretation of more subtle indications of patients' feelings. In still another setting, the pediatric unit, other demands are made on the nurse by virtue of the patient population, and as a result, the relation between beliefs and behavior is manifested somewhat differently.

Obviously, this research has not exhausted the various settings in which the relation between nurses' beliefs and behavior might profitably be studied. But the results of these three studies underscore the importance of considering situational variables in any general theory of nursing.

Implications for Nursing Research

Throughout this book we have suggested a number of potentially fruitful questions for future nursing research. At this point, however, we should like to mention two avenues of research that seem to be specifically promising. The first is based on our pilot investigation involving interviews of a small sample of highly empathic nurses. The second deals with an apparent paradox in nursing.

The Empathic Nurse

There is no simple way of describing or explaining the personal and professional development of an especially empathic nurse. It is much too complex a problem to be dealt with adequately in one very limited investigation. In this research, we feel that we have only scratched the surface of a very important problem, and the questions raised by this pilot investigation are far more significant than any tentative conclusions we might suggest. For example, how can nursing education foster and enhance a student's sense of commitment to nursing? Following the lead of the nurses we talked to, is a very demanding, highly structured, and rigorous course of training consistently related to the development of a sense of commitment and confidence? How can the conditions of nursing practice be designed to reinforce nurses' self-esteem and confidence? What are the factors in current practice that work against the development of professional self-esteem? How can nursing schools achieve an appropriate balance between emphasizing high level technical competence and recognizing the importance of interpersonal processes in nursing? Can we identify potentially important role models, and how can the impact of these role models be enhanced?

These are only a few of the questions raised by this study, and it is quite obvious that our research has resulted in many more questions raised than in answers even tentatively given. Addressing these questions in future research, however, may provide a systematic foundation for future advances in the education of nurses and the practice of nursing.

A Nursing Paradox

In the course of our research we have conducted several studies involving observations of nurses in interactions with patients. Our primary concern in these studies was the relation between a nurse's tendency to infer relatively high or low suffering and the ways she behaved in caring for patients. Although this relationship was the focus of our analysis, another aspect of the data was clearly apparent. Specifically, nursing behavior was focused much more often on the physical condition of patients rather than on their psychological distress. In terms of time during nurse-patient interactions, well over 80 percent of the time was consistently concerned with patients' physical condition; in terms of number of discrete nursing actions, over 75 percent focused on physical factors.

Thus, in our data at least, it is evident that much of hospital nursing care is devoted to physical rather than psychological factors. This observation is congruent with a great deal that has appeared in the nursing literature. Rarely are nurses told that they should pay attention to a patient's physical condition; it is simply assumed that a nurse will attend to the physical aspects of nursing care. But in countless articles, books, and speeches, nurses are exhorted to pay attention to a patient's psychological state. The writers of these articles, books, and speeches seem to assume that nurses neglect the psychological dimension of nursing. If our observations are at all representative of hospital nursing in the United States, this assumption is supported by our data. Indeed, nurses *do* pay much more attention to patients' physical function than to their psychological distress.

Previous efforts to correct this apparent imbalance seem to be based largely on the proposition that nurses need to be sensitized to patients' psychological distress, and if this sensitization is achieved, nurses will focus more attention on the psychological aspects of nursing care. However, our data on nurses' reactions to suffering clearly contradict this point of view. By and large, nurses *are* aware of patients' psychological distress. In study after study we have found that for the majority of patients, nurses consistently infer a greater degree of psychological distress than physical pain. As a matter of fact, we have discovered that over the course of nursing education, inferences of physical pain decrease, while inferences of psychological distress increase. Therefore it is clear from our data that, in general, nursing education is highly effective in sensitizing prospective nurses to the psychological distress likely to be experienced by patients. The problem, then, is not one of increasing nurses' awareness of the psychological dimension of nursing care. For the most part, by the time a nurse graduates and begins practice, he or she has already been sufficiently sensitized in this direction.

If nurses are indeed aware of patients' psychological distress, how can we account for the fact that a relatively small proportion of nursing behavior actually focuses on psychological care? A possible explanation rests on a consideration of situational factors, rather than the sensitivities of nurses. If one observes the typical hospital setting, it is apparent that the situation itself emphasizes almost exclusively a patients' physical condition. This is reflected in the well-established routines of nursing care. Almost all of these routines concern the physical dimension of nursing care. A nurse routinely evaluates, for example, a patient's temperature, pulse, and respiration; routinely records laboratory tests, medications, and anything else relevant to the patient's physical functioning and treatment. But while nursing administrators may from time to time encourage their nursing staff to be sensitive to psychological factors, consideration of these psychological factors is rarely incorporated into the daily routines of nursing care. Instead, the psychological dimension, though often cited as of prime importance in the nursing literature and during a nurse's education, is often relegated to almost incidental status in the formal routines of hospital care.

We come, then, to a central paradox in nursing. Nurses are abundantly aware of, sensitive to, and concerned with the psychological distress of their patients. On the other hand, at least in hospital settings, situational demands to focus primarily on the patient's physical condition are often so compelling that a nurse's concern with the psychological dimension of care must be slighted. Thus, the nurse may find herself in an apparent paradox. As a result of education, professional reading, and other personal and professional experiences, he or she has been sensitized to the psychological aspect of patient suffering. But the situation in which the nurse may work often demands an emphasis on physical care to a degree that may exclude realistic opportunities to deal with a patient's psychological distress.

An additional factor suggested to us by a number of nurses we have interviewed during this research concerns the techniques available to nurses for dealing effectively with patients' psychological distress. In discussing their professional education, these nurses felt well-prepared to respond to patients' pain with a variety of pain-relief measures. But at the same time, they felt ill-prepared to deal with patients' psychological distress under the conditions they face in hospital practice. In most instances, they felt, there was simply not enough time to use the psychotherapeutically based techniques they had been introduced to in their nursing education. Because of demands on their time and other responsibilities to fulfill, they could not engage in a therapeutically oriented nurse-patient interaction that required concentrated attention to one patient for extended periods of time.

At this stage, we cannot evaluate the legitimacy of these claims. Nevertheless, they suggest the possibility that nurses' relative inattention to the psychological distress of their patients may be, in part, a consequence of the lack of effective nursing techniques that are appropriate and practical in typical hospital settings.

These speculations suggest two interrelated avenues of nursing research. First, how can the hospital situation be changed systematically to encourage, rather than discourage, nursing attention to the psychological dimension of patient suffering? And second, what practical, realistic techniques are available, or can be developed, to deal effectively with patients' psychological distress under the actual conditions of hospitalization? In our opinion, both of these problems represent major areas of research for the continued improvement of nursing care.

References

Baer, E., Davitz, L. J., and Lieb, R. "Inferences of Physical Pain and Psychological Distress in Relation to Verbal and Nonverbal Patient Communication." *Nursing Research* 19 (1970): 388–392.

Barron, A. "The Effects Varied Nursing Approaches Have on Patients' Complaints of Pain: A Clinical Experiment." Unpublished Master's thesis, Yale University, 1964.

Beecher, H. K. "The Measurement of Pain." *Pharmacological Reviews* 9 (1957): 59–209.

Beecher, H. K. *Measurement of Subjective Responses.* New York: Oxford University Press, 1959.

Berblinger, K. W. "Influence of personalities on Drug Therapy." *American Journal of Nursing* 59 (1959): 1130–1132.

Blitz, B. and Dinnerstein, A. J. "Effects of Different Types of Instructions on Pain Parameters." *Journal of Abnormal Psychology* 93 (1968): 276–280.

Bochnak, M. A. "The Effect of Automatic and Deliberative Process of Nursing Activity on the Relief of Patients' Pain: A Clinical Experiment." Unpublished Master's thesis, Yale University, 1961.

Byrne, D. "The Repression-Sensitization Scale: Rationale, Reliability, and Validity." *Journal of Personality* 29 (1961): 334–349.

Chambers, W. G. and Price, G. G. "Influence of Nurse Upon Effects of Analgesics Administered." *Nursing Research* 16 (1967): 228–233.

Chapman, W. P. "Measurements of Pain Sensitivity in Normal Control Subjects and Psychoneurotic Subjects." *Psychosomatic Medicine* 6 (1944): 252.

Chapman, W. P. and Jones, C. M. "Variations in Cutaneous and Visceral Pain Sensitivity in Normal Subjects." *Journal of Clinical Investigations* 23 (1944): 81–91.

Clark, W. C. "Pain Sensitivity and the Report of Pain: An Introduction to Sensory Decision Theory." *Anesthesiology* 40 (1974): 272–287.

Clausen, J. and King, H. E. "Determinants of the Pain Threshold on Untrained Subjects." *Journal of Psychology* 30 (1950): 229–306.

Cohen, R. "The Effects of Specific Emotional Support on Anxiety Levels Prior to Electroconvulsive Therapy." *Nursing Research* 19 (1970).

Copp, L. A. "The psychology and philosophy of suffering." Unpublished paper presented at the Eighteenth Annual Cooperative Studies in Mental Health and Behavioral Science of Veterans Administration. New Orleans, 1973.

Copp, L. A. "The Spectrum of Suffering." *American Journal of Nursing* 74 (1974): 491–495.

Critchley, M. "Some Aspects of Pain." *British Medical Journal* 2 (1934): 891–896.

Davitz, L. J. and Davitz, J. R., "Nurses' Inferences of Suffering—Progress Report." (Unpublished report, NU00496) (1974) Division of Nursing, Department of Health Education, and Welfare.

Davitz, L. J. and Davitz, J. R. "How do Nurses Feel when Patients Suffer?" *American Journal of Nursing* 75 (1975): 1505–1510.

Davitz, L. J. and Pendleton, S. H. "Nurses' Inferences of Suffering. Study 1. Cultural Differences." *Nursing Research* 18 (1969a): 100–103.

Davitz, L. J. and Pendleton, S. H. "Nurses' Inferences of Suffering. Study 2. Clinical Specialties." *Nursing Research* 18 (1969b): 103–105.

Davitz, L. J. and Pendleton, S. H. "Nurses' Inferences of Suffering. Study 3. Patient Diagnosis." *Nursing Research* 18 (1969c): 104–105.

Davitz, L. J. and Pendleton, S. H. "Nurses' Inferences of Suffering. Study 4. Patient Characteristics." *Nursing Research* 18 (1969d): 105–107.

DeAugustinis, J., Isani, R. S., and Kumler, F. R. "Ward study: The Meaning of Touch in Interpersonal Communication, in S. Burd and M. Marshall." *Some Clinical Approaches to Psychiatric Nursing.* New York: The Macmillan Co., 1963.

Dichter, E. "A Psychological Study of the Hospital-Patient Relationship: what the patient really wants from the hospital. *Modern Hospital* 83 (1954): 54–55.

Diers, D., Schmidt, L. McBride, B., and Kette, L. D. "The Effect of Nursing Interaction on Patients in Pain." *Nursing Research* 21 (1972): 419–428.

Duff, R. S. (1972) and Hollingshead, A. B. *Sickness and Society.* New York: Harper and Row Publishers, 1968.

Dumas, R. G. and Leonard, R. C. "Effect of Nursing on the Incidence of Post-operative Vomiting." *Nursing Research* 12 (1963) 12–15.

Elder, R. G. "What is the Patient Saying?" *Nursing Forum* 2(1) (1963): 25–37.

Gelfand, S. "The Relationship Between Experimental Pain Tolerance and Pain Threshold." *Canadian Journal of Psychology* 18 (1964): 36–42.

Golub, S. and Reznikaff, M. "Attitudes Toward Death." A Comparison of Nursing Students and Graduate Nurses." *Nursing Research* November-December 1971.

Graham, L. E. and Conley, E. M. "Evaluation of Anxiety and Fear in Adult Surgical Patients." *Nursing Research* 20 (1971): 113–122.

Hall, K. R. L. and Stride, E. "The Varying Response to Pain in Psychiatric Disorders: A Study in Abnormal Psychology. *British Journal of Medical Psychology* 27 (1954): 48–60.

Hallstrom, B. J. "Contact Comfort: Its Application to Immunization Injections." *Nursing Research* 17 (1968).

Hamburger, M. "Realism and Consistency in Early Adolescent Aspirations and Expectations." Unpublished doctoral dissertation, Columbia University, 1958.

Hammond, K. R. "Clinical Inference in Nursing." *Nursing Research* 15 (1966a): 236–243.

Hammond, K. R. "Clinical Inference in Nursing." *Nursing Research* 15 (1966b): 330–336.

Hammond, K. R. "Clinical Inference in Nursing." *Nursing Research* 15 (1967): 38–45.

Hardy, J., Wolff, H., and Goodell, H. *Pain Sensations and Reactions.* New York: Hafner Publishing Company, 1952.

Hays, J. S. "Analysis of Nurse-Patient Communications." *Nursing Outlook* 14 (1966): 32–35.

Hays, J. S. and Larson, K. H. Interaction with Patients. New York: Macmillan Company, 1963.

Healy, K. M. "Does Preoperative Instruction Make a Difference?" *American Journal of Nursing* 68 (1968): 62–67.

Jacox, A. and Stewart, M. "Relation of Psychosocial Factors and Type of Pain." Mimeographed Report. University of Iowa, 1973.

Jarasuh, M. B., Rhymes, J. R., and Leonard, R. C. "An experimental test of the importance of communication skill for effective nursing" *Social Interaction and Patient care,* J. K. Shipper, Jr., and R. C. Leonard (eds.). Philadelphia: J. B. Lippincott Company, 1965, 110–120.

Johnson, B., Johnson, J. E., and Dumas, R. G. "Problem of Uncontrolled Situational Variables." *Nursing Research* 19 (1970).

Johnson, M. and Martin, H. D. "A Sociological Analysis of the Nurse's Role." *American Journal of Nursing* 58 (1958): 373–377.

Jourard, S. M. "Bedside manner." *American Journal of Nursing* 60 (1960): 63–66.

Keele, K. D. "A physician looks at pain." In *Pain: Clinical and Experimental Perspectives,* Matisyohu Weisenberg (ed.). Saint Louis: C. V. Mosby Company, 1975.

Keller, C. M. *The Relationship of Anxiety Changes and an Information Owing Experience.* New York University doctoral dissertation. 1965.

Kennard, M. A. "Responses to Painful Stimuli of Patients with Severe Chronic Painful Conditions." *Journal of Clinical Investigations 31* (1952): 245–252.

Kyle, Sister M. Willa. "The Nurse's Approach to the Patient Attempting to Adjust to Inoperable Cancer. *Effective Therapeutic Communications in Nursing* (Convention Clinical Sessions, No. 8). New York: American Nurses' Association 1964.

Lambert, W. E., Libman, E., and Poser, E. G. "The Effect of Increased Salience of a Membership Group on Pain Tolerance." *Journal of Personality* 28 (1960): 350–357.

Lasagna, L. C. "The clinical measurement of pain." *Annals of New York Academy of Science* 86 (1960): 28–29.

Lenburg, C. B., Glass, H. P., and Davitz, L. J. "Inferences of Physical Pain and Psychological Distress in Relation to the Stage of Patient's Illness and Occupation of the Perceiver." *Nursing* Research 19 (1970): 392–398.

Lenburg, C. B., Burnside, H. and Davitz, L. J. "Inferences of Physical Pain and Psychological Distress in Relation to Length of Time in the Nursing Education Program." *Nursing* Research 19 (1970): 399–401.

Lester, D., Getty, C. and Kneisl, C. R. "Attitudes of Nursing Students and Nursing Faculty Toward Death." *Nursing Research* 23: (1974), 50–53.

Loan, W. and Dundee, J. "The clinical assessment of pain." *Practitioner* 198 (1967): 759–768.

McBride, M. B. "Pain and Effective Nursing Practice." *American Nursing Clinical Sessions.* New York: Appleton-Century-Crofts, 1967, 75–82.

McCaffery, M. *Nursing Management of the Patient with Pain.* Philadelphia: J. B. Lippincott Company, 1972.

McCaffery, M. and Moss, F. "Nursing Intervention for Bodily Pain." *American Journal of Nursing* 68 June 1967: 1224–1227.

May, W. T. and Ilardi, R. L. "Value Changes in College Students." *College Student Journal,* November 1973.

Meehan, J. P., Stoll, A. M., and Hardy, J. D. "Cutaneous Pain Threshold in Native Alaskan Indian and Eskimos. *Journal of Applied Psychology* 6 (1954): 397–400.

Melzack, R. "The perception of pain." *Scientific American* 204 (1961): 41–49.

Merskey, H. "Psychological aspects of pain." *Postgraduate Medical Journal* 44 (1968): 297–306.

Ministry of Health and Welfare. *A Brief Report on Public Health Administration in Japan.* Ministry of Health and Welfare, Japanese Government, 1972.

Moody, P. M. "Attitudes of Cynicism and Humanitarianism in Nursing Students and Staff Nurses. *Journal of Nursing Education* 12: (1973), 9–13.

Moss, F. T. and Meyer, B. "Effects of Nursing Interactions Upon Pain Relief in Patients. *Nursing Research* 15 (1966): 303–306.

Newton, M. E., Hunt, W. E., McDowell, W., and Hanken A. F. *A Study of Nurse Action in Relief of Pain.* Columbus: The Ohio State University of Nursing, 1966.

Nikkari, J. G. *Freshman-to-Senior Personality Change in Basic Collegiate Student Nurses as Compared to Changes in Females in a Liberal Arts College in a Large Midwestern State University.* Ann Arbor: The University of Michigan, 1969.

Notermans, S. L. H. and Tophoff, M. M. "Sex Difference in Pain Tolerance and Pain Perception. *Pain: Clinical and Experimental Perspectives,* M. Weisenberg (ed.). St. Louis: C. V. Mosby Company, 1975.

Orlando, A. J. *Dynamic Nurse-Patient Relationship; Function; Process and Principles.* New York: G. P. Putnam's Sons, Inc., 1961.

Parisen, M. P., Rich, R., and Jackson, Jr. C. W., "Suitability of the Subjective Stress Scale for Hospitalized Subjects." *Nursing Research* 18 (1969): 529–533.

Petrie, A. *Individuality in Pain and Suffering.* Chicago: University of Chicago Press, 1967.

Putt, A. M. "One Experiment in Nursing Adults with Peptic Ulcers." *Nursing Research* 19 (1970).

Schmid, N. J. and Schmid, D. T. "Nursing Students' Attitudes Toward the Alcoholic." *Nursing Research* May-June 1973.

Skipper, J. K. "Communication and the Hospitalized Patient. *Social Interaction and Patient Care,* J. K. Skipper and R. C. Leonard (eds.). Philadelphia: J. B. Lippincott and Company, 1965, 61–82.

Stein, R. F. "The Student Nurse: A Study of Needs, Roles, and Conflicts, Part 1." *Nursing Research* July-August 1969.

Sternbach, R. A. and Tursky, B. "Ethnic Differences Among Housewives in Psychophysical and Skin Potential Responses to Electric Shock." *Psychophysiology* 1 (1965): 241–246.

Sullivan, H. S. *The Interpersonal Theory of Psychiatry.* New York: W. W. Norton, 1953.

Sullivan, R. "Examination of Criteria Used by Nurses in the Assessment of the Patient in Pain." Unpublished research project, St. Louis University, 1974.

Swartz, P. "Pain Scaling and the Influence of Sex and Personality on the Pain Response." Unpublished thesis, University of Rochester, New York, 1951.

Vando, A. "A Personality Dimension Related to Pain Tolerance." Unpublished doctoral dissertation, Columbia University, 1969.

Yeaworth, R. C., Kapp, F. T., and Winget, C. "Attitudes of Nursing Students Toward the Dying Patient." *Nursing Research* 23: (1974), 20–24.

Zborowski, M. People in Pain. California: Jossey Bass, 1969.

Appendix

The Standard Measure of
Inferences of Suffering Questionnaire

INSTRUCTIONS

Each of the items in this booklet contains a brief description of a patient. Please read the description of each patient, and then judge the degree of physical pain or discomfort and the degree of psychological stress the patient is probably experiencing. Indicate your judgments about each patient by checking the appropriate places on the two rating scales for each item.

Remember, there are no right or wrong answers. We are only interested in your judgments. Do the ratings as quickly as you can. Don't sit and think for a long time about any one item. Read the description of each patient and quickly size up the case. Then, on the basis of your first reaction to the case, check off the two rating scales, indicating how much physical pain or discomfort and how much psychological distress <u>you feel</u> the patient is experiencing.

		None	Little	Mild	Mod-erate	Great	Severe	Very Severe
1. Tripping on an uneven pavement block, Louise Crane, seventy years of age, fell and sustained a fractured femur. In traction at the moment, surgery is planned.	Physical Pain, Discomfort:	1	2	3	4	5	6	7
	Psycholog-ical Distress	1	2	3	4	5	6	7
2. Concerned about the appearance of a mole on her upper left arm, thirty-two year old Elizabeth Burdine decided to have the lesion removed in the doctor's office. The pathology report was negative.	Physical Pain, Discomfort:	1	2	3	4	5	6	7
	Psycholog-ical Distress	1	2	3	4	5	6	7
3. Thirty-six year old Gladys Lee stumbled and fell on the sidewalk, sustaining an abrasion of the hand. When the injury was not attended to, an abscess developed which required incision and drainage. She is to care for the hand through soaking and make an appointment to have the hand checked in a few days.	Physical Pain, Discomfort:	1	2	3	4	5	6	7
	Psycholog-ical Distress	1	2	3	4	5	6	7
4. Because of a persistent cough and a lingering cold, John Caldwell, age forty, was advised to consult a physician. His condition was diagnosed as broncho-pneumonia requiring hospitalization.	Physical Pain, Discomfort:	1	2	3	4	5	6	7
	Psycholog-ical Distress	1	2	3	4	5	6	7
5. While standing on a kitchen chair to reach a high shelf, Nancy Lynch, forty years old, slipped and fractured her right arm. X-rays indicated a frac-tured radius. The arm was placed in a cast, and now, after six weeks, the cast will be removed.	Physical Pain, Discomfort:	1	2	3	4	5	6	7
	Psycholog-ical Distress	1	2	3	4	5	6	7
6. "I expect something to happen to me. I feel I am seeing every-thing through a new awareness." Forty-one year old Howard Madison reflected his sense of foreboding and feelings of a brighter, clearer world during an intake interview.	Physical Pain, Discomfort:	1	2	3	4	5	6	7
	Psycholog-ical Distress	1	2	3	4	5	6	7

		None	Little	Mild	Mod-erate	Great	Severe	Very Severe
7. After a series of tests and examinations, Catherine Kent, forty-two years of age, was hospitalized with thrombophlebitis. Therapeutic measures include anticoagulants and bedrest.	Physical Pain, Discomfort:	1	2	3	4	5	6	7
	Psychological Distress	1	2	3	4	5	6	7
8. Undergoing an annual physical examination, Florence Tully, forty-two years of age was informed that she had a low grade systolic murmur. She has been hospitalized for a series of conclusive tests.	Physical Pain, Discomfort:	1	2	3	4	5	6	7
	Psychological Distress	1	2	3	4	5	6	7
9. Merle Lombard was rushed to the hospital by her mother after this nine year old child fell from a tree-house platform. X-rays indicated a fractured femur, and she has remained at the hospital in traction pending surgery.	Physical Pain, Discomfort:	1	2	3	4	5	6	7
	Psychological Distress	1	2	3	4	5	6	7
10. During a routine psychological test at his school, seven year old Austin Barett appeared troubled and concerned. When asked to arrange a series of blocks according to size and color, he insisted "they have sharp edges," and the "bright colors" bothered him.	Physical Pain, Discomfort:	1	2	3	4	5	6	7
	Psychological Distress	1	2	3	4	5	6	7
11. The general fatigue and behavior of seven year old Madeline Rankin concerned her parents. Seen by a pediatrician, she was admitted to the hospital with a possible diagnosis of leukemia. A complete diagnostic testing program is underway.	Physical Pain, Discomfort:	1	2	3	4	5	6	7
	Psychological Distress	1	2	3	4	5	6	7
12. Concerned about his frequent colds, William Hampton, seventy years old, went to a family doctor. Bronchopneumonia was diagnosed. Mr. Hampton was hospitalized and placed on antibiotic therapy.	Physical Pain, Discomfort:	1	2	3	4	5	6	7
	Psychological Distress	1	2	3	4	5	6	7

	None	Little	Mild	Mod-erate	Great	Severe	Very Severe
13. Concerned about his difficulties standing on his feet for any period of time, forty-one year old Martin Downes was examined by his doctor. Thrombophlebitis was diagnosed. Currently he is in the hospital being treated with anticoagulant drugs while on complete bedrest. — Physical Pain, Discomfort:	1	2	3	4	5	6	7
Psychological Distress	1	2	3	4	5	6	7
14. While pruning a hedge near his daughter's home, Edward Dennis injured his hand. At the insistence of his daughter, he finally saw a doctor. An incision and drainage of the abscess was performed in the office, and the seventy-two year old man was told to soak his hand and return in three days. — Physical Pain, Discomfort:	1	2	3	4	5	6	7
Psychological Distress	1	2	3	4	5	6	7
15. Concerned about a general malaise and an overall feeling of "not being himself," George James, forty years of age, consulted a doctor. Preliminary examination indicated a possibility of leukemia, and he is currently hospitalized undergoing a diagnostic work-up. — Physical Pain, Discomfort:	1	2	3	4	5	6	7
Psychological Distress	1	2	3	4	5	6	7
16. Because of increasing irritability over minor concerns and a general feeling of oversensitivity, Roberta Brower, seventy-two years of age, felt she should seek help from her family physician. — Physical Pain, Discomfort:	1	2	3	4	5	6	7
Psychological Distress	1	2	3	4	5	6	7
17. After leaving work, Ray Christopher, sixty-four years old, stumbled on an uneven sidewalk and fractured his femur. Surgery is planned. — Physical Pain, Discomfort:	1	2	3	4	5	6	7
Psychological Distress	1	2	3	4	5	6	7

		None	Little	Mild	Mod-erate	Great	Severe	Very Severe
18. Struggling with a toy, five year old Maureen Ferguson hurt her right hand. An abscess developed which the pediatrician incised and drained during an office visit. Maureen's mother was instructed how to soak the child's hand, and to be sure to bring her back to see the doctor in three days.	Physical Pain, Discomfort:	1	2	3	4	5	6	7
	Psychological Distress	1	2	3	4	5	6	7
19. While attempting to change a flat tire on his car, Frank Jordan, thirty-nine years of age, stumbled and struck his arm against the metal jack. The break was set in a cast which remained on the arm for six weeks. He is due to have the cast taken off in a day or so.	Physical Pain, Discomfort:	1	2	3	4	5	6	7
	Psychological Distress	1	2	3	4	5	6	7
20. At the suggestion of a pediatrician, a mole from five year old Joey Herter's right arm was surgically removed in the doctor's office. The pathology report was negative.	Physical Pain, Discomfort:	1	2	3	4	5	6	7
	Psychological Distress	1	2	3	4	5	6	7
21. Observing that Timothy Barnes, a nine year old fourth grader, could not remain seated any length of time and frequently appeared upset by the other children, his teacher sent him to the school nurse. This behavior had occurred with great frequency during the past week.	Physical Pain, Discomfort:	1	2	3	4	5	6	7
	Psychological Distress	1	2	3	4	5	6	7
22. Six year old James Stone was admitted to the hospital. His mother explained that the pediatrician noticed a heart murmur in a routine office examination, and he wanted James to have a complete series of tests.	Physical Pain, Discomfort:	1	2	3	4	5	6	7
	Psychological Distress	1	2	3	4	5	6	7

		None	Little	Mild	Mod-erate	Great	Severe	Very Severe
23. A number of self-concerns about how she was feeling prompted Marcia Claxton, thirty-eight years of age, to check her condition with a doctor. After a preliminary examination and a possible diagnosis of leukemia, hospitalization was deemed necessary for further testing.	Physical Pain, Discomfort:	1	2	3	4	5	6	7
	Psychological Distress	1	2	3	4	5	6	7
24. Eight year old Nancy Sloan had a mole excised from her arm the day before yesterday. She did not require hospitalization, and the biopsy report was negative.	Physical Pain, Discomfort:	1	2	3	4	5	6	7
	Psychological Distress	1	2	3	4	5	6	7
25. Bobby Simpson's mother is bringing him to an orthopedist to have a cast taken off his arm. A month and a half ago, Bobby, a kindergartner, fell from a Jungle Gym in the school playground and sustained a fracture of his right radial bone.	Physical Pain, Discomfort:	1	2	3	4	5	6	7
	Psychological Distress	1	2	3	4	5	6	7
26. Barbara King, forty years of age, told the nurse that many things were disturbing her. She continually worried about the future. Objects appeared to her to be much brighter and clearer than she had ever before experienced.	Physical Pain, Discomfort:	1	2	3	4	5	6	7
	Psychological Distress	1	2	3	4	5	6	7
27. In accordance with his company's requirement, Frederick Britt, age thirty-nine reported for an annual physical examination. The company physician noticed a heart murmur and has requested further tests.	Physical Pain, Discomfort:	1	2	3	4	5	6	7
	Psychological Distress	1	2	3	4	5	6	7
28. Jack Walters, thirty-three, had an excision of a mole from his lower arm done two days ago. The pathology report came back negative.	Physical Pain, Discomfort:	1	2	3	4	5	6	7
	Psychological Distress	1	2	3	4	5	6	7

	None	Little	Mild	Mod-erate	Great	Severe	Very Severe
29. Aware of his growing sense of irritability and general nervous tension at work, George Abbott, forty-four years of age, decided to check out his condition with his personal physician.	Physical Pain, Discomfort:	1	2	3	4	5	6	7
	Psychological Distress	1	2	3	4	5	6	7
30. Stumbling on an icy step, seventy-one year old Charlotte Timmons sustained a fractured left radial bone. Her arm was placed in a cast which has been on for about seven weeks. Her physician has decided that it can now be removed.	Physical Pain, Discomfort:	1	2	3	4	5	6	7
	Psychological Distress	1	2	3	4	5	6	7
31. A series of colds prevented nine year old Lisa Roberts from attending school regularly. As she was unable to get rid of a cough, she was taken to the pediatrician who had the child hospitalized for bronchopneumonia.	Physical Pain, Discomfort:	1	2	3	4	5	6	7
	Psychological Distress	1	2	3	4	5	6	7
32. Marian Benedict injured her hand and the resulting infection concerned her. She went to her doctor who performed an I and D in the office. The seventy-four year old woman is to soak her hand and to return to the physician's office in three days.	Physical Pain, Discomfort:	1	2	3	4	5	6	7
	Psychological Distress	1	2	3	4	5	6	7
33. Seventy-four year old Ernest Trew returned to his doctor's office for a biopsy report on a mole which had been excised from his upper right arm several days previously. The pathology report was negative.	Physical Pain, Discomfort:	1	2	3	4	5	6	7
	Psychological Distress	1	2	3	4	5	6	7
34. Waiting for her turn to be tested, Melanie Stillman, a fourth grader, told the school psychologist that the room light was disturbing. "Everything stands out and bothers me." She complained of feeling "funny" in her stomach.	Physical Pain, Discomfort:	1	2	3	4	5	6	7
	Psychological Distress	1	2	3	4	5	6	7

		None	Little	Mild	Mod-erate	Great	Severe	Very Severe
35. At the insistence of his family doctor, seventy-two year old Henry Marshall has entered the hospital for a complete series of diagnostic studies. An office examination suggested the possibility of leukemia.	Physical Pain, Discomfort:	1	2	3	4	5	6	7
	Psycholog-ical Distress	1	2	3	4	5	6	7
36. Retired, Chester Wilcox, age seventy-two, takes the precaution of having annual check-ups. He was notified at his last physical of the presence of a low grade systolic murmur. A diagnostic work-up has been scheduled.	Physical Pain, Discomfort:	1	2	3	4	5	6	7
	Psycholog-ical Distress	1	2	3	4	5	6	7
37. Jimmy Falconer, a ten year old boy, caught his finger in a jammed bike gear. An abscess developed which required incision and drainage. The pediatrician told Jimmy's mother how to soak the wound, and instructed her to bring the boy back to see him in a few days.	Physical Pain, Discomfort:	1	2	3	4	5	6	7
	Psycholog-ical Distress	1	2	3	4	5	6	7
38. Sixty-six year old Austin Beasly was informed that he had no alternative but to be hospitalized. Diagnosed as having thrombophlebitis, therapy which included bedrest and anticoagulant drugs was begun immediately.	Physical Pain, Discomfort:	1	2	3	4	5	6	7
	Psycholog-ical Distress	1	2	3	4	5	6	7
39. "I'm upset, and it's not my usual way," reported Wilma Gray, sixty-seven years of age, to a nurse during an intake interview. She worried, it seemed, about so much. The future, her life--all bothered her. She also said she hadn't changed her glasses, but objects seemed particularly clear to her. "I'm really frightened about the future."	Physical Pain, Discomfort:	1	2	3	4	5	6	7
	Psycholog-ical Distress	1	2	3	4	5	6	7

		None	Little	Mild	Mod-erate	Great	Severe	Very Severe
40. Mary Williams, sixty-eight years of age, was notified that a biopsy report was negative. A few days before, her physician had excised a lower arm lesion in an office visit.	Physical Pain, Discomfort:	1	2	3	4	5	6	7
	Psycholog-ical Distress	1	2	3	4	5	6	7
41. Jane Patterson, sixty-nine years of age, underwent a routine physical examination prior to obtaining additional insurance. A low grade systolic murmur was noted, and she was told hospital-ization was necessary in order for her to have a complete check-up.	Physical Pain, Discomfort:	1	2	3	4	5	6	7
	Psycholog-ical Distress	1	2	3	4	5	6	7
42. Lea Hamilton is impatiently waiting for her turn to see the doctor. According to this forty-five year old woman, she has felt high-strung and moody, which she says is not typical of her usual behavior.	Physical Pain, Discomfort:	1	2	3	4	5	6	7
	Psycholog-ical Distress	1	2	3	4	5	6	7
43. Fatigue, repeated colds, and a persistent cough prompted thirty-four year old Beth Frawley to seek treatment. Bronchopneu-monia was diagnosed and immediate hospitalization required.	Physical Pain, Discomfort:	1	2	3	4	5	6	7
	Psycholog-ical Distress	1	2	3	4	5	6	7
44. Complaining of discomfort in her left leg, sixty-seven year old Marie Cunningham made an appointment with her family doctor. The examination indicated thrombophlebitis. Hospitalization was necessary, and she is now being treated with anticoagulant therapy and bedrest.	Physical Pain, Discomfort:	1	2	3	4	5	6	7
	Psycholog-ical Distress	1	2	3	4	5	6	7

		None	Little	Mild	Mod-erate	Great	Severe	Very Severe
45. Complaining of general fatigue and malaise, seventy-one year old Rose Walker decided to see her family physician. Examination indicated a need for complete tests to rule out the possibility of leukemia.	Physical Pain, Discomfort:	1	2	3	4	5	6	7
	Psycholog-ical Distress	1	2	3	4	5	6	7
46. In traction pending surgery, eleven year old James Foreman sustained a fractured femur when his bike skidded on a wet road and he lost control.	Physical Pain, Discomfort:	1	2	3	4	5	6	7
	Psycholog-ical Distress	1	2	3	4	5	6	7
47. Currently on bedrest and receiving anticoagulant therapy, twelve year old William Post was hospitalized with a diagnosis of thrombophlebitis. His parents took him for an examination following the boy's repeated insistence that his "legs hurt."	Physical Pain, Discomfort:	1	2	3	4	5	6	7
	Psycholog-ical Distress	1	2	3	4	5	6	7
48. Routinely undergoing an annual physical required by the school, ten year old Jill Cox was found by her pediatrician to have a heart murmur. The physician recommended a thorough hospital examination.	Physical Pain, Discomfort:	1	2	3	4	5	6	7
	Psycholog-ical Distress	1	2	3	4	5	6	7
49. Seventy year old Shirly Adams ascribed her continual bouts of colds to the severity of the winter. However, at her family's insistence she did see a doctor who prescribed anti-biotic therapy and insisted she be hospitalized for broncho-pneumonia.	Physical Pain, Discomfort:	1	2	3	4	5	6	7
	Psycholog-ical Distress	1	2	3	4	5	6	7
50. Hospitalized and in traction as a result of a fall on an icy street, thirty-nine year old Joan Lawrence has been hospi-talized. Within a few days she'll be having surgery for the fractured femur.	Physical Pain, Discomfort:	1	2	3	4	5	6	7
	Psycholog-ical Distress	1	2	3	4	5	6	7

		None	Little	Mild	Mod-erate	Great	Severe	Very Severe

51. Jerome Fleming, thirty-eight years of age, was concerned about the swelling and pain in his hand from an injury he had received at work a week previously. He went to the office clinic and an abscess was incised and drained. After soaking the hand regularly for the next few days, he is due to have the hand checked.

	Physical Pain, Discomfort:	1	2	3	4	5	6	7
	Psychological Distress	1	2	3	4	5	6	7

52. Seventy-three year old Harvey Carpenter customarily followed a routine pattern. Recently, however, he has complained of feeling "edgy" and any suggestion made to him is reacted to with great irritation. The slightest change in schedule makes him nervous.

	Physical Pain, Discomfort:	1	2	3	4	5	6	7
	Psychological Distress	1	2	3	4	5	6	7

53. Concerned about their daughter's complaints of discomfort in her legs, the parents of twelve year old Janet Richards took her for an examination. Throbophlebitis was diagnosed, and Janet entered the hospital to begin treatment which consisted of bedrest and anticoagulants.

	Physical Pain, Discomfort:	1	2	3	4	5	6	7
	Psychological Distress	1	2	3	4	5	6	7

54. Richard Wylie, seventy-two years of age, slipped on an icy pavement six weeks ago. Since that time his fractured arm has been in a cast which his doctor has indicated will be ready to come off in the next day or so.

	Physical Pain, Discomfort:	1	2	3	4	5	6	7
	Psychological Distress	1	2	3	4	5	6	7

55. Noticing Monica Slater's moody and fretful behavior over the last several days, the fifth grade teacher sent the child to see the school nurse.

	Physical Pain, Discomfort:	1	2	3	4	5	6	7
	Psychological Distress	1	2	3	4	5	6	7

		None	Little	Mild	Mod-erate	Great	Severe	Very Severe
56. Benjamin Everett, sixty-five, told the nurse that he'd like an appointment with the doctor as soon as possible. Recently he's been feeling anxious "with waves of anxiety hitting me." He complained of worrying about the future and says he sees everything with great clarity.	Physical Pain, Discomfort:	1	2	3	4	5	6	7
	Psychological Distress	1	2	3	4	5	6	7
57. Six weeks ago, Laurie Jones, a second grader, lost her hold on the school monkey bars and broke her left humerus. An appointment has been made to have the cast removed from the arm.	Physical Pain, Discomfort:	1	2	3	4	5	6	7
	Psychological Distress	1	2	3	4	5	6	7
58. Upon admission to the emergency room following an auto accident, Lewis Knapp, thirty-six years old, was placed immediately in traction. Surgery will be necessary to repair a fractured femur.	Physical Pain, Discomfort:	1	2	3	4	5	6	7
	Psychological Distress	1	2	3	4	5	6	7
59. Eleven year old Stanely Overton seemed unable to shake a cough and cold. Examined by the family physician, his parents were informed that hospitalization and antibiotic therapy were necessary because of broncho-pneumonia.	Physical Pain, Discomfort:	1	2	3	4	5	6	7
	Psychological Distress	1	2	3	4	5	6	7
60. Admitted to the pediatric unit, Peter Goodwin, six years of age, is suspected of having leukemia. At present he is being examined and tested to rule out this possibility.	Physical Pain, Discomfort:	1	2	3	4	5	6	7
	Psychological Distress	1	2	3	4	5	6	7

Index

Index